Behavioral Health Care Delivery Following the Onset of the COVID-19 Pandemic

Utilization, Telehealth, and Quality of Care for Service Members with PTSD, Depression, or Substance Use Disorder

KIMBERLY A. HEPNER, CAROL P. ROTH, JESSICA L. SOUSA, TEAGUE RUDER, RYAN ANDREW BROWN, LAYLA PARAST, HAROLD ALAN PINCUS

Prepared for the Connected Health Branch, Clinical Support Division, Medical Affairs, Defense Health Agency
Approved for public release; distribution unlimited

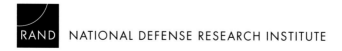 NATIONAL DEFENSE RESEARCH INSTITUTE

For more information on this publication, visit **www.rand.org/t/RRA421-3**.

About RAND

The RAND Corporation is a research organization that develops solutions to public policy challenges to help make communities throughout the world safer and more secure, healthier and more prosperous. RAND is nonprofit, nonpartisan, and committed to the public interest. To learn more about RAND, visit www.rand.org.

Research Integrity

Our mission to help improve policy and decisionmaking through research and analysis is enabled through our core values of quality and objectivity and our unwavering commitment to the highest level of integrity and ethical behavior. To help ensure our research and analysis are rigorous, objective, and nonpartisan, we subject our research publications to a robust and exacting quality-assurance process; avoid both the appearance and reality of financial and other conflicts of interest through staff training, project screening, and a policy of mandatory disclosure; and pursue transparency in our research engagements through our commitment to the open publication of our research findings and recommendations, disclosure of the source of funding of published research, and policies to ensure intellectual independence. For more information, visit www.rand.org/about/research-integrity.

RAND's publications do not necessarily reflect the opinions of its research clients and sponsors.

Published by the RAND Corporation, Santa Monica, Calif.
© 2023 RAND Corporation
RAND® is a registered trademark.

Library of Congress Cataloging-in-Publication Data is available for this publication.

ISBN: 978-1-9774-0863-1

Cover: U.S. Air Force photo/Heather Heiney.

About This Report

The COVID-19 pandemic, which was declared a public health emergency in February 2020, tested the resilience of the U.S. health care sector like no other disruption in recent history. At the pandemic's onset, the Military Health System (MHS) was already exploring options to expand its use of telehealth, including for behavioral health (BH) conditions. Relying on administrative data on BH visits from the period immediately following the onset of the pandemic and an equivalent period in 2019, RAND researchers conducted preliminary analyses of changes in care delivery in the MHS for posttraumatic stress disorder, depression, and substance use disorder. The findings provide insights about changes in BH care utilization patterns, the use of telehealth, and the effects on the quality of BH care provided to service members. The resulting recommendations can help guide the MHS as it takes steps to expand the use of telehealth, improve health care access and quality, and increase its resilience in the face of future disruptions.

The research reported here was completed in December 2021 and underwent security review with the Defense Office of Prepublication and Security Review before public release.

RAND National Security Research Division

This research was sponsored by the Defense Health Agency and conducted within the Forces and Resources Policy Center of the RAND National Security Research Division (NSRD), which operates the National Defense Research Institute (NDRI), a federally funded research and development center sponsored by the Office of the Secretary of Defense, the Joint Staff, the Unified Combatant Commands, the Navy, the Marine Corps, the defense agencies, and the defense intelligence enterprise.

For more information on the RAND Forces and Resources Policy Center, see www.rand.org/nsrd/frp or contact the director (contact information is provided on the webpage).

Acknowledgments

We gratefully acknowledge the support of our project sponsor, Robert Ciulla, Connected Health Branch, Clinical Support Division, Medical Affairs, Defense Health Agency. We also appreciate the ongoing support of Anju Bhargava, Fuad Issa, Kate McGraw, and staff at the Connected Health and the Psychological Health Center of Excellence. We appreciate the valuable insights we received from Shira Fischer and Jan A. Lindsay. We addressed their constructive critiques as part of RAND's rigorous quality assurance process to improve the quality of this report. We thank Lauren Skrabala for her contributions to sections of this report. Finally, we thank Laurence Ma for her assistance in preparing this report and Jessica Sousa for overseeing human subjects and regulatory approvals for the project.

Summary

The Military Health System (MHS) was already taking steps to expand the integration of telehealth for the treatment of behavioral health (BH) conditions when the COVID-19 pandemic began in early 2020. The MHS, like the rest of the U.S. health care sector, adopted protocols to allow physical distancing and keep service members and providers safe. The public health crisis represented a potential major disruption in care for service members who required treatment for such BH conditions as posttraumatic stress disorder (PTSD), depression, and substance use disorder (SUD). How did patterns of BH care utilization change following the onset of the pandemic? Under what circumstances and to what extent was telehealth incorporated into BH treatment? Were there declines in the quality of care that service members received during this period?

This report presents a preliminary examination of changes in BH care delivery in the MHS following the onset of the pandemic, including BH care utilization patterns, use of telehealth, and the quality of BH care. We compared BH care in two six-month periods: April–September 2019, prior to the onset of the pandemic, and April–September 2020, following pandemic-related restrictions on care delivery. Drawing on the findings from these preliminary analyses, we developed recommendations to help the MHS continue to improve BH care and mitigate the potential effects of the pandemic, with a focus on implications for the ongoing integration of telehealth.

Research Approach

Our data sample included active-component and National Guard/reserve service members who were enrolled in TRICARE and had at least one health care encounter with a diagnosis of PTSD, depression, or SUD in fiscal years 2018–2020. Specific analyses had narrower eligibility criteria.

We assessed changes in BH care delivery following the onset of the pandemic and associated pandemic-related restrictions (April–September 2020) by making comparisons with an equivalent pre-pandemic period (April–September 2019). Using MHS administrative records, we identified monthly patterns in BH care utilization for service members with PTSD, depression, or SUD over each six-month period to detect changes in BH care delivery among service members who received treatment from direct care providers at military treatment facilities (MTFs) and from private-sector providers contracted by TRICARE. Specifically, we compared the number of BH visits received, BH visit settings (i.e., primary care versus specialty care), and the number of treatment visits received (i.e., for psychotherapy or medication management). We also identified cohorts of service members with a new episode of PTSD, depression, or SUD in the first three months of our observation periods and summarized their use of BH care in the three months after initiating care. We employed a similar approach to assessing the use of telehealth for these BH conditions and supplemented our descriptive analyses with statistical modeling.

To detect potential changes in the quality of BH care following the onset of the pandemic, we selected 21 measures that aligned with clinical practice guidelines for PTSD, depression, and SUD. We used these measures to assess the quality of BH care before and after the onset of the pandemic in three domains: initial care for new treatment episodes, medication management, and transitions of care.

Key Findings

We drew the following conclusions from these preliminary analyses of BH care utilization patterns, changes in the use of telehealth, and the quality of BH care that service members received following the onset of the COVID pandemic.

Pandemic-Related Restrictions Prompted Changes in Behavioral Health Care Delivery

We observed several differences between the April–September 2019 and April–September 2020 periods in terms of monthly BH care utilization (across all modalities, including in-person and telehealth visits) by BH diagnosis, treatment type, provider type, and source of care:

- There were 50,000 *fewer* BH visits in 2020 than in the equivalent period in 2019, but overall monthly patterns of care were not significantly different.
- Patterns of care utilization for SUD, specifically, were significantly different between the two periods, indicating *fewer* visits in 2020 than in 2019. There were also significantly *fewer* group psychotherapy visits overall.
- The majority of BH visits for service members with PTSD, depression, or SUD occurred in direct care settings (i.e., at MTFs), but there were significantly *fewer* monthly BH visits in 2020 than in 2019. The opposite was true in private-sector care settings (i.e., where care is delivered by TRICARE-contracted providers): There were significantly *more* monthly BH visits in 2020 than in 2019.
- Service members had significantly *fewer* BH visits with primary care providers and social workers during the 2020 pandemic period than in 2019, but we did not detect a difference for other BH providers.
- *Fewer* service members initiated treatment for all three conditions in 2020 than in 2019. However, those who initiated treatment for PTSD or depression had significantly *more* BH visits. For all three conditions, those who received individual psychotherapy had *more* visits than those who did so in 2019.

The drop in the number of BH visits could have been because service members delayed care or because of a lack of available appointments (Jowers, 2020). Clinic closures and challenges associated with rapid telehealth implementation with the onset of the pandemic also might have affected BH care utilization differently in direct and private-sector care settings. For example, prior RAND research suggests that many military providers found it challenging to deliver group psychotherapy via telehealth, and some elected to suspend sessions to support physical distancing during the pandemic (Hepner, Sousa, et al., 2021). However, the results regarding utilization must be interpreted with caution because it is unclear how pandemic-related restrictions affected care in terms of access (e.g., those who needed care received it) and timeliness (e.g., availability of appointments to those who received care).

Telehealth Use Increased Markedly After the Onset of the Pandemic but Varied by Type of Treatment

The pattern of telehealth and in-person BH visits differed significantly between 2019 and 2020.

- There were only around 7,000 telehealth visits (all modalities of telehealth) per month between April and September 2019, when BH care in the MHS was delivered primarily in person (93 percent). During this same period in 2020, there were approximately 42,000–59,000 telehealth visits for BH care, with the highest volume in April 2020 (67 percent of BH visits), soon after the pandemic's onset.
- In April 2020, 66 percent of individual psychotherapy and 75 percent of evaluation and management/medication management visits were conducted via telehealth. This share steadily declined over the remainder of the observation period, likely reflecting a return to in-person visits and an easing of pandemic-restrictions.
- The majority of direct care BH telehealth visits (83 percent) were coded as audio-only, whereas only 1 percent of private-sector care visits were. Prior RAND research indicates that direct care providers faced technological barriers to implementing video telehealth (Hepner, Sousa, et al., 2021). However, variations in provider coding guidance and practices could have resulted in data that did not clearly distinguish between video and audio-only visits. Therefore, it is unclear what proportion of coded telehealth visits relied on each modality.
- Most service members who initiated a new treatment episode of PTSD, depression, or SUD between April and June 2020 received a mix of in-person and telehealth BH visits in the three months after initiating care, rather than solely in-person or telehealth-based care.

There was variability in the definitions of telehealth modalities and related coding guidance for providers that the MHS and TRICARE issued, making it difficult to accurately assess the use of video versus audio-only telehealth. However, these findings provide useful insights into how telehealth in general was employed in different care settings and for different types of BH visits.

Behavioral Health Care Quality Was Largely Sustained or Improved Following the Onset of the Pandemic, Although Fewer Service Members Were Seen for PTSD, Depression, or SUD

We used 21 measures to evaluate the quality of BH care delivered to service members in April–September 2019 and April–September 2020. These measures provided insights about the quality of initial care, medication management, and transitions of care during these periods. Recommended care could have been delivered by any modality (i.e., in person or via telehealth).

- The quality of BH care was largely sustained or improved following the onset of the pandemic. Compared with the 2019 observation period, we detected little change in care quality on ten of 21 measures, and there were improvements on seven measures.
- Seven measures addressed initial care quality, and the MHS held steady or improved on six of them between 2019 and 2020. However, one measure declined: A smaller share of service members with a new SUD diagnosis received psychotherapy in 2020 than in 2019.
- The MHS also held steady or improved on six of eight measures addressing medication management. However, this was not the case for two measures: Fewer service members with PTSD or depression who initiated new medication treatment received a follow-up visit within 30 days.
- In terms of timely outpatient follow-up after care transitions, quality was similar or improved on five of six measures. Scores for follow-up after psychiatric hospitalization within 30 days, while high, were lower in 2020 than in 2019.
- These measure scores, including those that remained stable, varied widely in both years and across domains (ranging from 7 to 92 percent), suggesting several areas for improvement, particularly when it comes to the timely delivery of treatment or follow-up care.

Although fewer service members with PTSD, depression, or SUD were seen in the MHS in 2020, our data indicated that they generally received care of comparable quality to what they received in 2019, despite the challenges posed by the pandemic. It should be noted that we were unable to capture levels of unmet need in this study or assess how pandemic-related factors might have affected access to or the timeliness of care received.

Policy Implications

Although this research was preliminary, the findings highlight where the MHS might continue ongoing efforts to integrate telehealth into the high-quality BH care that service members receive, as well as opportunities for change, improvement, and future research.

Recommendation 1. Continue the Expanded Use of Telehealth for Behavioral Health Care and Monitor Care Quality

Our analyses highlighted a marked expansion in the use of telehealth following the onset of pandemic-related restrictions. The MHS was already taking steps to integrate telehealth into BH care delivery (U.S. House of Representatives, 2016; Pamplin et al., 2019), but the pandemic required a rapid, evolving response to ensure care availability and continuity (Mehrotra et al., 2020; MHS Communications Office, 2020; Pamplin et al., 2019; Uscher-Pines et al., 2020). Despite these challenges, our analyses suggest that the quality of BH care by most measures *did not decline* in 2020 and even *improved* in some areas. Although it is important to note that fewer service members received treatment in April–September 2020 than in the same period in 2019, these findings suggest that telehealth could support MHS efforts to improve BH care quality and access. Telehealth will also likely play an important role in preparedness for future disruptions in care—from pandemics to natural disasters. For these reasons, we recommend that the MHS continue to expand its use of telehealth, alongside efforts to monitor BH care quality and access on an ongoing basis, rather than reducing telehealth delivery to pre-pandemic levels.

Recommendation 2. Assess Behavioral Health Treatment Outcomes Among Service Members Who Receive Telehealth

We were not able to compare service members' treatment outcomes, such as symptom improvement, in the pre-pandemic and pandemic periods. Prior to the pandemic, providers collected data on patient symptoms using the Behavioral Health Data Portal (BHDP), a tool that proved difficult to adapt for telehealth visits. To help ensure continuity of symptom tracking and the accuracy of outcome monitoring, the MHS is preparing to update BHDP to allow providers to collect patient-reported measures remotely. Once the system is in place, the MHS could leverage the resulting data to examine the treatment implications of telehealth and its effect on patient outcomes.

Recommendation 3. Increase the Clarity of Telehealth Coding Guidance for Providers

We encountered challenges in our analyses as a result of ambiguity in the provider guidance for telehealth coding that the MHS and TRICARE circulated at the start of the pandemic. For example, there were variations in how telehealth modalities were defined and how they were subsequently coded by providers. As the MHS continues to explore telehealth expansion, standardized coding guidance for telehealth visits will be essential to monitoring the quality of care that service members are receiving.

Conclusions

The COVID-19 pandemic provided a lesson in resilience for the health care sector. The MHS was already exploring options to expand telehealth integration into BH care practices, and the preliminary analyses in this report support these efforts and can inform decisions about further telehealth adoption. If implemented appropriately, telehealth likely has an important role to play in strengthening military readiness and improving access to high-quality BH care for service members.

Contents

Figures and Tables

Figures

Tables

CHAPTER ONE

Introduction

The U.S. Department of Defense (DoD) aims to provide consistent, high-quality care to service members with behavioral health (BH) conditions through the Military Health System (MHS). The onset of the COVID-19 pandemic in 2020 prompted local and national restrictions on in-person care delivery that rapidly changed how the MHS provided treatment to service members with such conditions as posttraumatic stress disorder (PTSD), depression, and substance use disorder (SUD). Restrictions on in-person care delivery led to a marked increase in the use of telehealth to deliver care to service members who could no longer be seen in person safely. However, it remained unknown how patterns of care shifted during this time and how quality of care may have been affected. This report provides a preliminary examination of changes in BH care delivery following the onset of the pandemic, including the utilization of BH care, use of telehealth, and quality of BH care. To describe changes in patterns of care, we compared two six-month periods: April–September 2019, prior to the onset of the pandemic, and April–September 2020, following pandemic-related restrictions on care delivery. Drawing on findings from these preliminary analyses, we developed recommendations to help the MHS continue to improve care and mitigate the potential effects of the pandemic, with a focus on implications for ongoing integration of telehealth.

In this chapter, we provide an overview of the impact of the COVID-19 pandemic on BH care delivery in the MHS, the integration of telehealth into BH care delivery, and the importance of assessing the quality of BH care provided to service members.

COVID-19 and Behavioral Health Delivery in the MHS

Estimated prevalence rates of BH conditions among service members varied prior to the onset of the pandemic, but an analysis of available data reports published between 1985 and 2012 suggested that approximately 9–10 percent of service members had PTSD, 6–7 percent had depression, and 12–15 percent had alcohol use disorder (Cohen et al., 2015). Preliminary data suggest that pandemic-related stressors may have contributed to an increased need for BH care among both civilians and military personnel. Nationally representative surveys showed an increased prevalence of symptoms of depression (Ettman et al., 2020) and serious psychological distress (McGinty et al., 2020) among U.S. adults following the onset of the pandemic. A RAND study found that the prevalence of serious psychological distress in May 2020 was equal to that of the entire 12 months preceding the pandemic (Breslau et al., 2021). Subsequent research suggested that elevated rates of depression, substance use, and suicidal ideation persisted in civilian populations through September 2020 (National Center for Health Statistics, 2020; Czeisler et al., 2021; Holland et al., 2021; Vahratian et al., 2021). Preliminary survey data that relied on a nonrepresentative sample of service members showed that 18 percent of active-duty respondents reported new onset of anxiety or depressive symptoms after the start of the pandemic, and 15 percent reported worsened symptoms of a preexisting anxiety or depressive disorder (Strong, Akin, and Brazer, 2020).

Concurrent with this increase in BH needs, pandemic-related restrictions required a rapid shift away from in-person care (Mehrotra et al., 2020; Torous and Wykes, 2020). There was a risk of COVID-19 exposure among patients and providers alike, and efforts to promote physical distancing relied heavily on telehealth in many care settings (Mann et al., 2020). At the national level, the federal government announced temporary discretion for providers in Health Insurance Portability and Accountability Act (HIPAA) enforcement for good-faith use of less-secure telehealth platforms and allowed remote prescribing of controlled substances. The Centers for Medicare and Medicaid Services also agreed to cover audio-only and direct-to-home telehealth visits. These changes removed many of the constraints previously placed on telehealth delivery in civilian settings (see U.S. Department of Health and Human Services [DHHS], 2020; Drug Enforcement Administration, 2020; and Verma, 2020). Similar changes affected care provision for service members. The Defense Health Agency (DHA) released interim guidance on data security and privacy related to telehealth use in direct care settings in March and August 2020, and it published an interim final rule on TRICARE regulations in May 2020 to allow audio-only visits and facilitate telehealth use in private-sector settings (Cordts, 2020; Place, 2020; DoD, 2020). At the time of this writing in October 2021, DHA was continuing to develop formal policy guidance on acceptable uses for telehealth in the MHS after the end of the public health crisis, including which BH conditions or procedures are most appropriate for telehealth (Aker, 2021; Kime, 2020).

Integration of Telehealth in MHS Behavioral Health Care

In the MHS, *telehealth* is defined as "the use of telecommunications and information technologies to provide health assessment, diagnosis, treatment, consultation, education, and health-related information across distances" (MHS, undated). The term *telehealth* is often used synonymously with *virtual health* in the MHS. As defined by the MHS Virtual Health Clinical Integration Office, telehealth includes synchronous (real-time) videoconferencing visits between a provider and patient; asynchronous modalities, such as store-and-forward communication (electronic sharing of documents or images), remote patient monitoring, and other "terrestrial and wireless communications" (MHS, undated). The 2017 National Defense Authorization Act identified telehealth implementation as a top priority for the MHS (Pub. L. 114-328, 2016). Subsequent efforts by DHA to expand telehealth use within the MHS were numerous but focused mostly on individual initiatives to expand telehealth capabilities at selected military treatment facilities (MTFs) and military regional health care centers (Wheeler, 2021).

In the years preceding the COVID-19 pandemic, synchronous telehealth implementation in the MHS was largely limited to video visits between providers and patients located at MTFs (Madsen, Banaag, and Koehlmoos, 2021; U.S. Government Accountability Office, 2017). In most regions of the continental United States, telehealth was not regularly provided to service members in their homes (Luxton et al., 2015; Luxton et al., 2016). Telehealth use by private-sector providers contracted by TRICARE was also limited prior to the pandemic (U.S. Government Accountability Office, 2017; Wheeler, 2021). Although telehealth use within the MHS had increased in recent years, these increases seem to have occurred more quickly in private-sector settings than at MTFs (Madsen, Banaag, and Koehlmoos, 2021). One analysis of MHS telehealth services between 2006 and 2008 found that synchronous visits accounted for most of the increase in telehealth utilization in that period, but there was not an upswing in the use telehealth for mental health diagnoses until 2015 in private-sector settings and 2017 at MTFs (Madsen, Banaag, and Koehlmoos, 2021). A recent RAND study on access and quality of BH care for remote service members found that the proportion of service members with PTSD, depression, or SUD who had any synchronous telehealth visits during a six-month observation period was small (3 percent) (Hepner, Brown, et al., 2021). However, restrictions associated with the COVID-19 pandemic rapidly changed care delivery (Connolly et al., 2021; Mehrotra et al., 2021; Patel et al., 2020; Uscher-Pines et al., 2020). Beginning in April 2020, physical distancing requirements precipitated an immediate change in the way care was delivered at MTFs.

A more recent RAND report summarized the perspectives of 53 BH clinicians and administrators at ten MTFs on their experiences delivering care during the COVID-19 pandemic (Hepner, Sousa, et al., 2021). These staff described a dramatic transition from in-person care in the early months of the pandemic, a shift to audio-only visits, a combination of audio-only and video visits, or a suspension of care altogether. Changes were highly variable across MTFs. Most staff reported that they continued to see the most acute or highest-risk patients in person. Some expressed concern about using telehealth for service members with PTSD and SUD (nearly one-third and one-fifth, respectively), and half reported concerns about using telehealth with high-risk or acute patients. One-third of staff across all the MTFs in the study reported concerns about using telehealth with new patients. Additionally, one-quarter mentioned that group therapy sessions had stopped during the pandemic. Staff cited significant challenges associated with the expansion of telehealth: Many lacked the necessary equipment and broadband access for telehealth, while a "learning curve" was often mentioned in accounts of using telehealth platforms. Staff at most MTFs expressed frustration with unclear guidance, bureaucratic barriers, or a perceived lack of MTF or DHA support for telehealth. At the time of the interviews in July–October 2020, half of staff reported a return to more in-person care. In light of these findings, the report recommended that the MHS develop clear policy guidance on the appropriateness of telehealth use, implement a strategic plan to support technology and infrastructure, and provide clinical and technical training on the use of telehealth (Hepner, Sousa, et al., 2021).

Ensuring High-Quality Behavioral Health Care

The COVID-19 pandemic was associated with changes and restrictions on health care delivery, prompting an increased use of telehealth. It is essential to ensure that service members receive high-quality BH care, even with such changes in practice. Quality measures help assess whether care aligns with evidence-based clinical practice guidelines (CPGs) by indicating what percentage of service members have received care concordant with CPGs. Prior RAND research assessed the quality of BH care in the MHS for service members with PTSD, depression, and SUD (Hepner, Brown, et al., 2021) using measures based on U.S. Department of Veterans Affairs (VA)/DoD CPGs for these conditions (Hepner, Brown, et al., 2021; VA and DoD, 2015, 2016, 2017). The assessed domains of BH care included initial care, medication management, and transitions of care. The results of that study identified several strengths in how the MHS delivered care to service members with these diagnoses. For example, more than 75 percent of those with a new treatment episode (NTE) of PTSD or depression received psychotherapy or recommended medication treatment within four months. More than 70 percent of those with PTSD or depression who initiated new medication treatment received that medication for an appropriate duration. Furthermore, 93 percent of service members who were discharged from a psychiatric hospitalization had a follow-up visit with a mental health provider within 30 days, and 78 percent of those who were seen in an emergency department (ED) for a mental health reason received a follow-up visit within 30 days.

That study also identified areas for improvement. For example, less than 30 percent of service members with a PTSD or depression NTE received four psychotherapy visits or two evaluation and management (E&M) visits in the first eight weeks, and few with an SUD NTE initiated and engaged in SUD care (16 percent and 7 percent, respectively). Fewer than half of those with PTSD, depression, or SUD who initiated new medication treatment received a follow-up visit within 30 days. With respect to transitions of care, just 21 percent of service members who were seen in an ED for a substance use problem received a follow-up visit within 30 days (Hepner, Brown, et al., 2021).

One commonality across these results is the need for timely access to care, for both ongoing treatment and follow-up visits. Thus, the MHS needs to continue to take steps to ensure access and reduce barriers to BH care. That earlier RAND study also indicated that care was not consistent across different populations: Service members who lived in areas that were remote from MTF care received lower-quality care on several measures. The findings suggested that telehealth could be a mechanism to increase timely access to treatment and follow-up visits (Hepner, Brown, et al., 2021). Note that the recommendation to increase telehealth use was made prior to the pandemic. With the onset of the pandemic, many aspects of care delivery changed abruptly, and it was unknown whether the quality of care delivered declined because of these changes, which included a heavy reliance on telehealth.

Organization of This Report

In this report, we examine changes in BH care delivery for service members with PTSD, depression, or SUD following the onset of the pandemic, including BH care utilization patterns, use of telehealth, and quality, by comparing care in two six-month periods (April–September 2019 and April–September 2020). In Chapter Two, we provide an overview of our methodological approach. Chapters Three through Five present our findings related to BH care utilization patterns, use of telehealth, and quality of BH care, respectively. In Chapter Six, we summarize key findings and provide recommendations to help the MHS continue to improve BH care after the pandemic ends.

Four appendixes provide additional background on the data coding process, our analyses of BH care utilization, telehealth utilization, and the quality measures used in our study.

CHAPTER TWO

Methods

In this chapter, we describe the methods used for the analyses presented in this report. We summarize the data sources used and the criteria for identifying eligible active-component service members to include in our analyses. We also describe our approach to assessing utilization of BH services, use of telehealth for BH care, and the quality of care provided for PTSD, depression, and SUD. All study methods were approved by RAND's Institutional Review Board and the DHA Headquarters Human Research Protection Office.

Data Sources

We used several sources of administrative data to select eligible service members and to characterize aspects of their BH care, including patterns in their use of health care services, receipt of telehealth, and the quality of BH care they received. Table 2.1 lists the data files used in our analyses.

TABLE 2.1
Content of the Administrative Data Files Used in the Analyses

Content	Data Files
Outpatient services delivered at MTFs (direct care)	Comprehensive Ambulatory Professional Encounter Record (CAPER)
Inpatient services delivered at MTFs (direct care)	Standard Inpatient Data Record
Electronic health record outpatient data (direct care)	GENESIS Episodic Encounter
Electronic health record inpatient data (direct care)	GENESIS Basic Admission
Provider services delivered outside of MTFs (private-sector care)	TRICARE Encounter Data–Noninstitutional
Facility services delivered outside of MTFs (private-sector care)	TRICARE Encounter Data–Institutional
Dispensed medication (direct care and private-sector care)	Pharmacy Data Transaction Services
TRICARE enrollment, demographics	VM6 Beneficiary Level
Deployment history (September 2001–December 2020)	Contingency Tracking System–Deployments

The MHS delivers care to active-component service members through direct care, which is provided in MTFs, and private-sector care, which is delivered by civilian providers and is contracted and paid for by TRICARE. The administrative data files for these two forms of care came from the MHS Data Repository, a data source maintained by DHA. The files included records on all inpatient and outpatient health care encounters for TRICARE beneficiaries paid by TRICARE, either partially or in full. We de-duplicated and linked all records to the service member receiving the care. The detailed steps in this process, including variable names and codes, are documented elsewhere (Hepner et al., 2016).

Pre-Pandemic and Pandemic Comparison Periods

To assess changes in BH care delivery following the onset of the pandemic, we compared two six-month periods—prior to the onset of the pandemic (April–September 2019) and following pandemic-related restrictions on care delivery (April–September 2020). We selected a six-month observation period to allow an adequate period of care in which to apply several measures of BH care quality. We also determined that restrictions on in-person care had been implemented widely by April 2020 (Figure 2.1). We thus selected the same months (April–September) in both years to mitigate the effect of seasonal variations in BH care delivery.

FIGURE 2.1

Timeline of Analysis Periods and Contemporaneous Pandemic-Related Events

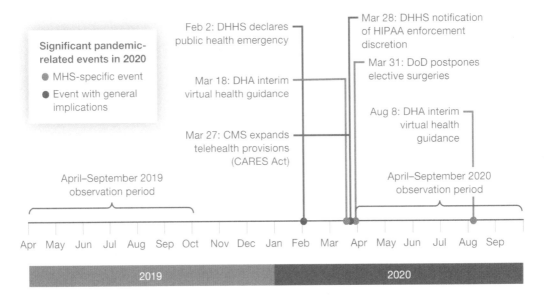

SOURCES: DHHS, 2020; DHA, 2020; DHHS, 2022; DoD, 2022; Centers for Medicare and Medicaid Services, 2020; Cordts, 2020.
NOTES: CMS = Centers for Medicare and Medicaid Services; CARES Act = Coronavirus Aid, Relief, and Economic Security Act.

Our primary analyses focused on comparing these two six-month periods. In some cases, we examined time frames outside of these two periods (e.g., 2018) to illustrate trends over longer periods and to frame our time-focused analyses. These analyses of extended periods are presented in the appendixes. We note that the analyses in this report are limited to treatment provided by the MHS. We were unable to characterize the level of unmet need in our two observation periods.

Study Eligibility Criteria

We identified service members who had at least one health care encounter with a diagnosis of PTSD, depression, or SUD during fiscal years (FYs) 2018–2020. We selected these diagnostic groups in collaboration with the study sponsor, prioritizing the potential impact on readiness if these conditions are not appropriately treated. To this population, we applied additional study eligibility criteria to identify service members who received care during the two study periods and to determine eligibility for inclusion in specific analyses, depending on the observation period of each analysis and whether the service member continued to meet the study criteria. The study eligibility criteria were as follows:

- *Service member status.* Eligible service members were 18–64 years old, in the active component or National Guard/reserves and not located overseas. Military retirees and family members were excluded.
- *Received care for PTSD, depression, or SUD.* Eligible service members had at least one encounter with a PTSD, depression, or SUD diagnosis (primary or secondary position). Eligible encounters included those delivered by direct care or private-sector care providers. Diagnosis codes for the study conditions are described elsewhere (Hepner, Brown, et al., 2021).[1]
- *Enrolled in MHS care.* Service members must have been enrolled in TRICARE during the entire period of study. Members who deployed or separated from military service were excluded.

Service members were eligible for inclusion in our analyses if they met these criteria, along with additional criteria specific to each analysis.

Analyses

As noted earlier, to assess changes in BH care delivery following the onset of the pandemic, we compared two six-month time periods—prior to the onset of the pandemic (April–

---

[1] Minor changes were made to the International Classification of Diseases, 10th revision (ICD-10), codes defining depression in this study: F0630, F39, and F4321 were deleted, and F338 was added.

September 2019) and following pandemic-related restrictions on care delivery (April–September 2020). We conducted analyses to compare BH care utilization patterns, use of telehealth, and quality of BH care between these two periods. The analyses focused on different populations of interest within our larger sample. Throughout this report, we provide both (1) a description of patterns observed (e.g., magnitude and direction) for the outcomes of interest and (2) results based on a statistical analysis of the significance (or lack thereof) of these observed patterns.

Utilization of Behavioral Health Care

We computed monthly utilization of BH care visits (i.e., associated with an ICD-10 F-code) during the six-month observation periods. We conducted utilization analyses at the month level. To be included in these analyses, service members needed to have at least one study diagnosis–related encounter during the month of interest, in addition to the criteria described earlier. Monthly utilization analyses included BH visits; visits with a primary diagnosis of PTSD, depression, or SUD; visits by source (i.e., direct versus private-sector care) and by setting (i.e., primary versus BH specialty care); and treatment visits received (i.e., psychotherapy, medication management). These analyses provided a snapshot of BH care delivered each month to service members with PTSD, depression, or SUD. We used regression models to examine whether there was a significant change in utilization from 2019 to 2020. These models used the number of visits per month as the outcome and included the following predictors: month indicators and an indicator for 2020 (versus 2019), where our test of interest assessed whether the regression coefficient for the 2020 indicator was significant. In presenting the results, we describe total utilization in each period (e.g., total number of BH visits in April–September 2019 versus April–September 2020) but note that significant testing compared the *patterns or trajectory of care over time* between the two periods rather than total visits in each period.

In addition, we identified three cohorts of service members with an NTE of PTSD, depression, or SUD during the first three months of the six-month observation periods (i.e., April–June 2019 and April–June 2020), and we observed their care during the three months following the initial visit for the NTE.[2] These analyses provided a summary of all BH care received by the cohorts of service members who initiated care for PTSD, depression, or SUD in the three months after the first visit. Specifically, we compared the total number of BH visits and the types of visits received (i.e., psychotherapy, medication management). We tested differences between the median number of visits using a two-sample median test based on a linear rank statistic.

---

[2] NTE for PTSD or depression was defined as a primary diagnosis and no encounters or medication treatment for the condition in the prior six months. NTE for SUD was defined as encounter with an SUD diagnosis with no SUD diagnosis-related encounter in the prior two months.

Use of Telehealth for Behavioral Health Care

We also examined the use of telehealth to deliver outpatient BH care in the early months of the pandemic (April–September 2020). We first describe the number of telehealth and in-person visits by month in the two studied periods. Then, for the six-month period in 2020, we describe the modalities of telehealth used, the percentage of visits that relied on telehealth by settings of care, and types of BH visits. We also describe the use of telehealth in direct and private-sector care. In addition, for the cohorts of service members with an NTE for PTSD, depression, or SUD, we describe the use of telehealth in the three months following the initiation of care.

Modalities of telehealth and how they are defined can vary (Center for Connected Health Policy, undated). Telehealth that involves real-time interaction is often referred to as *synchronous telehealth*. Prior to the COVID-19 pandemic, video visits were the most common type of synchronous telehealth, as Medicare and many commercial payers did not reimburse for audio-only visits (American Telemedicine Association, 2017; Verma, 2020; Volk et al., 2021). *Asynchronous telehealth* refers to a modality in which there is no real-time communication, such as the one-way transmission of medical information. This type of telehealth is often used to transmit images or patient test results and is used less often in BH care than in other specialties (Deshpande et al., 2009).

To define the modalities of telehealth for this study, we reviewed several sources of guidance for MHS providers addressing the different modalities of telehealth and the related coding used to document telehealth encounters (see Table A.1 in Appendix A). We found that the use of the terms *synchronous* and *asynchronous* and definitions in telehealth guidance for providers were not always consistent or precisely described. Synchronous telehealth was sometimes broadly defined as two-way communication in real time, with no requirement for video (i.e., seemingly inclusive of both audio-only and video modalities). In other cases, synchronous telehealth was specified as using both audio and visual telecommunication and was categorized separately from audio-only telehealth.

MHS guidance on the use of telehealth and its coding changed over time following the onset of the pandemic. These changes may have resulted in some inconsistencies among military providers in the way telehealth encounters were coded during our 2020 observation period. In developing our approach to coding telehealth encounters, we reviewed MHS and TRICARE coding guidance and consulted with telehealth subject-matter experts from DHA regarding definitions and coding of telehealth modalities.

Drawing on these sources of information, we categorized telehealth for our analyses as shown in the box on the following page, with the caveat that coding variations across providers and types of telehealth encounters might have affected the consistency with which telehealth visits in our data fell into these categories as defined. Specifically, the video synchronous category could include a mix of video and audio-only visits. See Appendix A for the coding algorithm we used to categorize BH telehealth encounters (Table A.2), as well as related telehealth modifiers and codes (Table A.3).

> **Telehealth Modalities**
>
> - *Video:* Synchronous (live), interactive telecommunication that includes audio and video.
> - *Audio only:* Synchronous (live), interactive audio-only communication using telephone or other audio-only technology.
> - *Asynchronous:* Storing, forwarding, and transmitting of medical information in one direction at a time.

Our analyses focused solely on outpatient BH visits in a population of service members with a diagnosis of PTSD, depression, or SUD and, therefore, do not represent all telehealth received by service members during the studied time periods. Furthermore, we excluded telehealth involving provider-to-provider consults, telehealth with inpatients or with patients in the ED, and patient-to-provider online or digital interactions (e.g., secure messaging, use of patient portal). In addition to descriptive analyses, we conducted significance testing to assess whether telehealth use differed between 2019 and 2020. Like the analyses of BH care utilization patterns, we used regression models to examine whether there was a significant change in the use telehealth and in-person care in these two periods. These models used the number of telehealth (or in-person) visits per month as the outcome and included the following predictors: month indicators and an indicator for 2020 (versus 2019), where our test of interest was assessing whether the regression coefficient for the 2020 indicator was significant.

Quality of Behavioral Health Care

We selected quality measures to assess the care received for PTSD, depression, and SUD during the two observation periods in both direct and private-sector care settings. We selected these process-of-care measures based on several criteria, including their use in prior research to assess the quality of BH care delivered by the MHS (Hepner et al., 2017; Hepner, Brown, et al., 2021; Hummer et al., 2021), their application requiring only administrative data, and our ability to apply the measures to a six-month observation period. The measures assess aspects of care related to initial care for NTEs, medication management, and transitions of care and are consistent with recommendations in the current VA/DoD CPGs for PTSD, depression, and SUD (Table 2.2) (VA and DoD, 2015, 2016, 2017). Details of the measures (overview, rationale for selection, and technical specifications) are reported elsewhere (Hepner, Brown, et al., 2021). We implemented measures that were endorsed by the National Quality Forum (NQF) according to specifications that were current as of 2018 (National Quality Forum, undated). All quality measures included in this study are process measures (i.e., they assess for receipt of recommended care). We were unable to include any outcome measures because use of the Behavioral Health Data Portal (BHDP), the MHS system to monitor patient-reported symptoms, declined following the onset of the pandemic. BHDP relied

TABLE 2.2

Quality Measures of Behavioral Health Care and Applicable Conditions

Measure	PTSD	Depression	SUD
Initial care			
Patients with an NTE who received any psychotherapy or any treatment with an SSRI/SNRI (PTSD) or antidepressant (depression) within the first 4 months	X	X	
Patients with an NTE for SUD who received any psychotherapy during the 6-month observation period			X
Patients with an NTE for PTSD or depression with 4 psychotherapy visits or 2 E&M visits within 8 weeks	X	X	
Patients with an NTE for AOD who received[a] • Initiation of AOD treatment within 14 days • Engagement of AOD treatment with 2 or more encounters within 30 days of initiation encounter			X
Medication management			
Patients with a newly prescribed medication with an adequate trial • PTSD: SSRI/SNRI for ≥60 days • Depression: antidepressant for 12 weeks[a]	X	X	
Patients with an NTE for AUD or OUD who received pharmacotherapy during the 6-month observation period • AUD: AUD pharmacotherapy • OUD: OUD pharmacotherapy			X
Patients with a newly prescribed medication with an E&M visit within 30 days • PTSD: SSRI/SNRI • Depression: antidepressant • AUD NTE: AUD pharmacotherapy • OUD NTE: OUD pharmacotherapy	X	X	X
Transitions of care			
Psychiatric inpatient hospital discharges with follow-up in[a] • 7 days • 30 days	X	X	X
ED discharges for MH or AOD with follow-up in[a] • MH: 7 days • MH: 30 days • AOD: 7 days • AOD: 30 days	X	X	X

NOTES: AOD = alcohol or other substance use disorder. This acronym is used rather than *SUD* when it appears in the original measure language. SSRI/SNRI = selective serotonin reuptake inhibitor/serotonin-norepinephrine update inhibitor. AUD = alcohol use disorder. OUD = opioid use disorder. MH = mental health.

[a] NQF-endorsed measure.

heavily on patient portals or tablets in waiting areas, making remote administration of measures for telehealth visits impractical.

We present descriptive findings for each quality measure applied, characterizing receipt of recommended care in 2019 and 2020. We conducted significance testing using chi-squared tests to compare quality measure scores by year.

Identification of Service Members for Inclusion in the Analyses

Figure 2.2 shows the selection process and eligibility criteria used to identify service members for the previously described analyses. We started with a base population of service members who met our initial eligibility criteria and had at least one encounter with a diagnosis of PTSD, depression, or SUD in the MHS administrative data for FYs 2018–2020. From that population, we identified those who met criteria for inclusion in each type of analysis during the two study periods.

FIGURE 2.2

Selection of Service Members with PTSD, Depression, or SUD for Inclusion in the Analyses

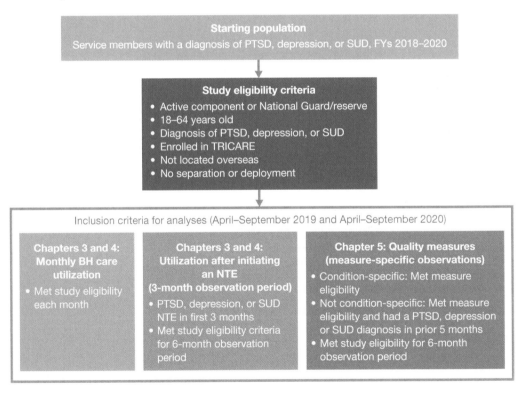

Accounting for Multiple Comparisons

Throughout this report, we present results from statistical analyses assessing the significance of differences or trends. To account for multiple comparisons, we note at the end of each chapter the total number of tests conducted and the number that would be expected to be significant by chance based on our alpha level of 0.05 used for testing.

Summary

Using administrative data, we selected service members with PTSD, depression, or SUD for analyses focused on two periods that corresponded to six months (April–September) in 2019 prior to the pandemic and the same six months in 2020 during the early months of the pandemic. Our analyses included monthly utilization of BH care during both observation periods. We also conducted analyses of BH care utilization over three months for cohorts of service members with an NTE of PTSD, depression, or SUD. We summarized the use of telehealth overall and by source of care, setting, and type of BH visit, as well as the proportion of telehealth to in-person care. Finally, we applied 21 measures to evaluate the quality of BH care delivered during both observation periods.

CHAPTER THREE

Utilization of Behavioral Health Care Following the Onset of the Pandemic

In this chapter, we compare BH care utilization patterns over a six-month period prior to the COVID-19 pandemic (April–September 2019) with an equivalent six-month period following the onset of the pandemic that saw the introduction of physical distancing restrictions (April–September 2020). We used these analyses to evaluate changes in outpatient BH care utilization patterns among service members with a diagnosis of PTSD, depression, or SUD following the onset of the pandemic. In the first half of the chapter, we examine overall patterns of behavioral health care utilization by month in 2019 versus 2020. In the second half of the chapter, we examine changes in utilization for cohorts of service members who initiated an NTE for PTSD, depression, or SUD in 2019 versus 2020 over a three-month period of care. The analyses in this chapter include all coded BH visits in MHS direct care and private-sector care data and do not distinguish the modality of care (i.e., they include both in-person and telehealth BH visits). The box below provides an overview of the key findings presented in this chapter.

Overview of BH Care Utilization Patterns, April–September 2019 and April–September 2020

- There were more than 50,000 fewer BH visits in the six-month observation period in 2020 than during the same six months in 2019, but the pattern of care utilization between the two periods was not significantly different.
- In comparing the two periods, there were significantly *fewer* monthly BH visits delivered at MTFs and significantly *more* monthly BH visits delivered by private-sector providers in 2020 compared with 2019.
- Service members received *fewer* group therapy visits in the observed months of 2020 than in 2019. *Fewer* BH visits were provided by social workers and primary care providers.
- Fewer service members initiated treatment for PTSD, depression, or SUD in 2020 compared with 2019. Service members who initiated treatment for PTSD or depression in 2020 received significantly *more* visits in the three months after initiating treatment than in 2019. We did not observe this difference for SUD.

Utilization of Behavioral Health Care

In this section, we examine monthly differences in BH visits, BH visits by target diagnosis, source of care (direct care versus private-sector care), care setting and provider type, and types of visits (e.g., psychotherapy, medication management) in 2019 versus 2020 (e.g., April 2019 versus April 2020, May 2019 versus May 2020, and so on).

Monthly Behavioral Health Visits

Figure 3.1 shows BH visits associated with any BH diagnosis. There were more than 50,000 fewer BH visits in the six-month observation period in 2020 than during the same six months in 2019 (557,386 versus 610,991), but care utilization patterns in these periods were not significantly different. For example, in April 2020, shortly after the implementation of pandemic-related restrictions, there were nearly 20,000 fewer BH visits compared with April 2019 (87,805 versus 107,255). Figure B.1 in Appendix B presents total monthly BH visits for service members with PTSD, depression, and SUD in 2018–2020.

Service members included in our analyses were required to have a diagnosis of PTSD, depression, or SUD, so we also examined the number of monthly visits for each of these target

FIGURE 3.1

Monthly BH Visits Among Service Members with PTSD, Depression, or SUD, 2019 and 2020

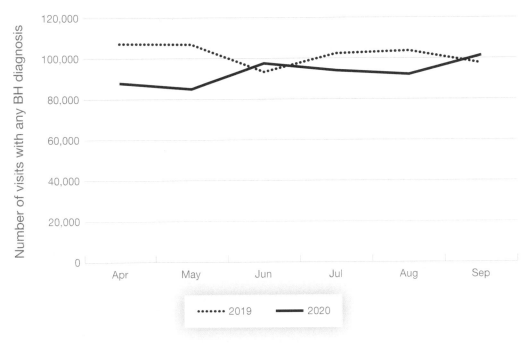

NOTES: Outpatient visits by month coded with a BH diagnosis in any position. Includes both in-person and telehealth visits. Results of the regression model were not significant.

diagnoses (Figure 3.2). Overall, the patterns observed for number of visits for these primary diagnoses were similar to the pattern for all BH diagnoses (Figure 3.1). However, our findings indicate some variability by diagnosis. Of these three target diagnoses, the largest numbers of visits were associated with a depression diagnosis in both six-month periods (164,526 in 2020 and 169,305 in 2019). Monthly visits with a primary depression diagnosis in June and September 2020 *exceeded* those in the same months in 2019. The pattern for visits associated with a primary PTSD diagnosis was similar but with a smaller monthly volume (123,484 total visits in 2020 and 128,338 in 2019). Regression analyses comparing the patterns of visits between the two years indicate that the differences were not statistically significantly for PTSD and depression.

In contrast, total monthly visits associated with a primary SUD diagnosis showed a larger decrease than for PTSD or depression in the six-month observation period in 2020 compared with 2019 (from 156,520 visits in 2019 to 128,723 in 2020). Although visit numbers for SUD recovered by September 2020 to a level comparable with that in September 2019, visit numbers in all six months observed in 2020 never exceeded the monthly numbers in

FIGURE 3.2

Monthly Visits with a Primary Target Diagnosis Among Service Members with PTSD, Depression, or SUD, 2019 and 2020

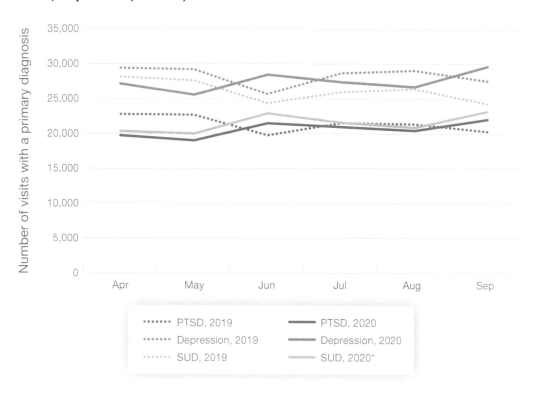

NOTES: Outpatient visits by month coded with the target diagnosis (PTSD, depression, or SUD) in the primary position. Includes both in-person and telehealth visits. * $p < 0.05$.

the same months of 2019. Regression analyses comparing the patterns of visits between the two years indicate that differences were significantly different for SUD ($p < 0.05$). Again, these decreases in monthly visits were not reflective of seasonal variation. Figures B.2–B.4 in Appendix B show monthly BH visits with a primary diagnosis of PTSD, depression, or SUD in 2018–2020.

While most BH visits were delivered at MTFs (i.e., direct care) in both years, a lower proportion of BH visits were delivered at MTFs in 2020 (72.9 percent) compared with 2019 (80.2 percent) relative to visits delivered by TRICARE-contracted private-sector providers. Figure 3.3 shows the extent to which the change in monthly BH visits differed for direct care compared with private-sector care. There were significantly *fewer* monthly BH visits delivered at MTFs in the six-month observation period in 2020 following the onset of the pandemic than in 2019 ($p < 0.05$; total visits April–September 2019: 489,950; 2020: 406,243). In contrast, there were significantly *more* monthly BH visits delivered by TRICARE-contracted private-sector providers ($p < 0.01$; total visits 2019: 121,041; 2020: 151,143).

FIGURE 3.3

Monthly BH Visits Among Service Members with PTSD, Depression, or SUD, by Source of Care, 2019 and 2020

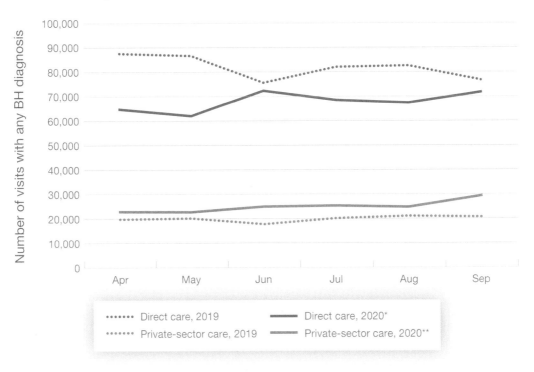

NOTES: Outpatient visits by month coded with a BH diagnosis in any position. Includes both in-person and telehealth visits. * $p < 0.05$, ** $p < 0.01$.

Visits by Setting and Provider Type

Most outpatient BH visits occurred in BH specialty care settings in both 2019 and 2020 (Figure 3.4). Although there were fewer total BH specialty care visits in 2020 than in 2019, the pattern of visits over time between the two periods was not significantly different (results not shown; 2019: 513,160; 2020: 478,518). Similarly, there were fewer total BH visits in primary care settings following the onset of the pandemic in 2020 than in the period prior to the pandemic, but the pattern between the two periods did not differ significantly (not shown; 2019: 62,082; 2020: 50,723).

Figure 3.5 shows BH care utilization by provider type. Regression analyses comparing the two periods suggest that utilization patterns differed for social workers and primary care practitioners but did not differ for psychiatrists or clinical psychologists. Specifically, there were significantly *fewer* monthly BH visits delivered by social workers and primary care practitioners following to onset of the pandemic ($p < 0.05$).

FIGURE 3.4

Monthly BH Visits Among Service Members with PTSD, Depression, or SUD, by Care Setting, 2019 and 2020

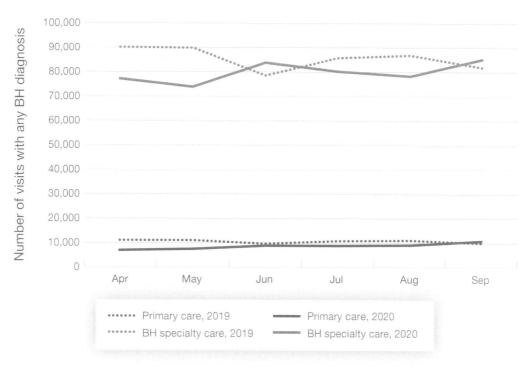

NOTES: Outpatient visits by month coded with a BH diagnosis in any position. Includes both in-person and telehealth visits. Results of the regression model were not significant for primary care or BH.

FIGURE 3.5

Monthly BH Visits Among Service Members with PTSD, Depression, or SUD, by Provider Type, 2019 and 2020

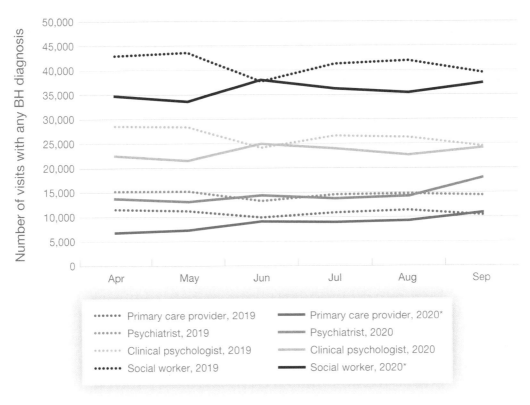

NOTES: Outpatient visits by month coded with a BH diagnosis in any position. Includes both in-person and telehealth visits. $^* p < 0.05$.

Psychotherapy and Evaluation and Management Visits

Specific types of psychotherapy (e.g., cognitive behavioral therapy) and specific types of medication (e.g., antidepressants) are the recommended first-line treatment options for PTSD, depression, and SUD (VA and DoD, 2015, 2016, 2017). We examined patterns of individual and group psychotherapy visits, along with E&M visits that can include medication management, shown in Figure 3.6. Although the total number of individual psychotherapy visits was slightly higher in 2020 compared with the same months in 2019, the difference in utilization patterns between the two periods was not statistically significant (results not shown; 2019: 290,980; 2020: 303,779). In contrast, the pattern of group therapy visits was significantly different, with fewer group psychotherapy visits in the period following the onset of the pandemic ($p < 0.001$; 2019: 64,593; 2020: 21,231). Although we observed fewer E&M/medication management visits in 2020 than in 2019, the pattern of visits was not significantly different (not shown; 2019: 165,875; 2020: 146,116).

FIGURE 3.6

Monthly Psychotherapy and E&M/Medication Management Visits Among Service Members with PTSD, Depression, or SUD, 2019 and 2020

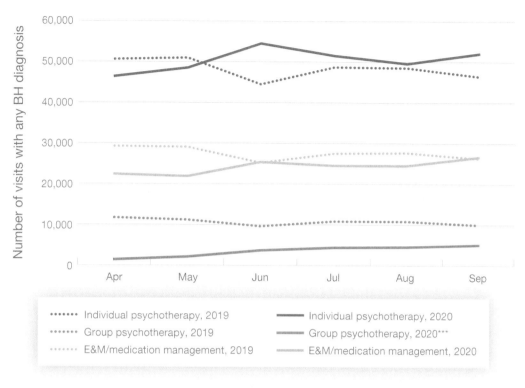

NOTES: Outpatient visits by month coded with a BH diagnosis in any position. Includes both in-person and telehealth visits. *** $p < 0.001$.

Utilization After Initiating a New Treatment Episode

In the prior analyses, we presented monthly BH care utilization patterns for service members with PTSD, depression, or SUD who received BH care during the observed months. In the following analyses, we identified three cohorts of service members with an NTE for PTSD, depression, or SUD during the first three months of the six-month observation periods (i.e., April–June 2019, April–June 2020) and observed their care in the three months following the initial visit. These analyses show BH care utilization for a cohort of service members over an equivalent period of three months following the initial visit. We compared the number of BH visits received, the setting for these BH visits (i.e., primary versus specialty care), and the number of treatment visits received (i.e., psychotherapy, medication management) in 2019 versus 2020. Overall, approximately 2,600 fewer service members initiated treatment for these target diagnoses following the onset of the pandemic than in the pre-pandemic period (Figure 3.7). This difference was more pronounced for depression and SUD. It is unclear how

FIGURE 3.7

Service Members Who Initiated a New Treatment Episode for PTSD, Depression, or SUD, April–June 2019 and 2020

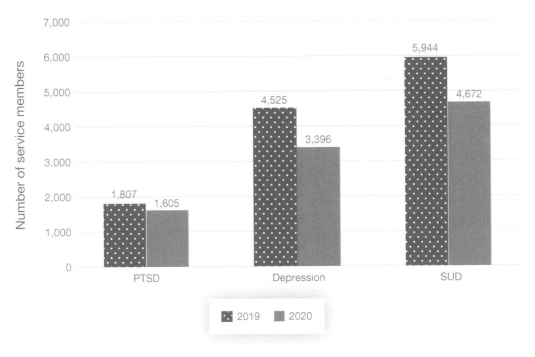

NOTES: Service members who initiated an NTE in April–June 2019 and April–June 2020. An NTE is initiated by a diagnosis-related encounter following a period of no diagnosis-related encounters.

pandemic-related restrictions affected the number of service members with an NTE who received care in 2020 versus 2019 (e.g., access issues, severity of symptoms).

We compared the median number of BH visits in the three months after initiating an NTE for PTSD, depression, or SUD. The pattern of findings differed across diagnoses. Service members in the NTE cohort who had their initial visit with a PTSD diagnosis received significantly *more* visits in 2020 than in 2019 (Table 3.1; $p < 0.001$). This was true for visits with a primary diagnosis of PTSD and for visits with any BH diagnosis. Similarly, service members initiating an NTE for depression received significantly *more* BH visits in 2020 ($p < 0.01$), although visits with a primary depression diagnosis did not differ. In contrast, the pattern of visits for service members initiating treatment for SUD did not differ between 2019 and 2020. Where there were significant differences but medians were equal, the distribution of the number of visits above and below the median was different between the two periods (see Table B.1 in Appendix B). Service members who initiated care for depression had a median of five visits (any BH diagnosis) within three months in both 2019 and 2020. However, 22 percent had four to six visits, and 41 percent had seven or more visits in 2020, compared with 25 percent and 38 percent, respectively, in 2019. It is unknown how pandemic-related restrictions might have affected the number of visits provided to those who received care (e.g., less

TABLE 3.1

BH Visits Within Three Months After Initiating a New Treatment Episode, 2019 and 2020

Cohort	Median Number of Visits	
	April–September 2019	April–September 2020
PTSD	(*n* = 1,807)	(*n* = 1,605)
Any BH diagnosis, any position***	5	6
PTSD diagnosis, primary position***	3	4
Depression	(*n* = 4,525)	(*n* = 3,396)
Any BH diagnosis, any position[a]**	5	5
Depression diagnosis, primary position	2	2
SUD	(*n* = 5,944)	(*n* = 4,672)
Any BH diagnosis, any position	6	6
SUD diagnosis, primary position	2	2.5

NOTES: Visits include both in person and telehealth. ** $p < 0.01$, *** $p < 0.001$.

[a] Although the medians are equal, the distribution of visits above and below the median are different for the two time periods.

overall demand for appointments allowing for increased timeliness of care for those who received care).

We also assessed median BH treatment visits (psychotherapy or E&M/medication management) for a subset of NTE cohorts—those with at least one visit of the designated type (Table 3.2). Across all three target conditions, service members who initiated an NTE and received at least one individual psychotherapy visit received significantly *more* individual psychotherapy visits following the onset of the pandemic than in 2019. In contrast, we did not observe a difference for group therapy visits. Service members initiating an NTE for PTSD received significantly more E&M/medication management visits within three months in 2020 compared with the same period in 2019. Median visits did not differ significantly for service members with depression or SUD. Where there were significant differences but medians were equal, the distribution of the number of visits above and below the median was different between the two periods (see Table B.2 in Appendix B). Service members initiating care for PTSD had a median of four individual psychotherapy visits within three months in 2019 and 2020. However, 32 percent had seven or more visits in 2020, compared with 23 percent in 2019. Service members initiating care for PTSD had a median of three individual psychotherapy visits within three months in 2019 and 2020. However, 24 percent had seven or more visits in 2020, compared with 17 percent in 2019.

TABLE 3.2

Target Diagnosis-Related Visits Within Three Months for Service Members with a New Treatment Episode for PTSD, Depression, or SUD, 2019 and 2020

Cohort and Visit Type	April–September 2019		April–September 2020	
	Had at Least One Visit (%)	Median Number of Visits	Had at Least One Visit (%)	Median Number of Visits
PTSD	(n = 1,807)		(n = 1,605)	
Individual psychotherapy[a]***	72.8	4	75.8	4
Group psychotherapy	4.8	2	2.1	2
E&M/medication management**	46.2	1	41.7	2
Depression	(n = 4,525)		(n = 3,396)	
Individual psychotherapy[a]***	58.9	3	58.5	3
Group psychotherapy	4.8	2	1.3	2
E&M/medication management	54.8	2	51.2	2
SUD	(n = 5,944)		(n = 4,672)	
Individual psychotherapy***	53.4	3	56.1	4
Group psychotherapy	28.5	5	13.5	4
E&M/medication management	46.3	2	45.4	2

NOTES: Median outpatient visits coded with the target diagnosis in any position in the three months after initiating a new treatment episode among service members who received at least one visit with the designated visit type. Visits include both in person and telehealth. ** $p < 0.01$, *** $p < 0.001$.

[a] Although the medians are equal, the distribution of visits above and below the median are different for the two observation periods.

Summary

We compared monthly utilization patterns of BH care provided to service members with PTSD, depression, or SUD between April–September 2019 and the same period in 2020. In addition, we compared service members' overall BH care utilization in the three months after initiating an NTE for PTSD, depression, or SUD in 2019 versus 2020. Although we observed several changes in BH care delivery following the onset of the pandemic, these preliminary analyses do not identify the reasons for these differences. For example, some decreases in BH care utilization could be a result of a lack of access to appointments, lack of adequate clinical staffing, a reduced need for care, or an inability to provide remote access to care. The following highlights from these analyses capture the results of our examination of monthly BH care utilization before and following the onset of the pandemic and differences in sources of BH care, numbers of treatment visits, and care utilization after initiating an NTE:

- **Monthly utilization:** There were more than 50,000 fewer BH visits in the six-month observation period in 2020 than during the same six months in 2019 (557,386 versus 610,991), but the pattern between the two periods was not significantly different. The pattern of monthly visits for SUD was significantly different between 2019 and 2020, indicating fewer visits in all months of the 2020 observation period; the monthly pattern did not differ for PTSD and depression.
- **Source of care:** More BH visits were delivered at MTFs (i.e., direct care) in both 2019 (80.2 percent) and 2020 (72.9 percent) than by TRICARE-contracted private-sector providers. It appears that the pandemic affected MTF care differently from private-sector care. There were significantly *fewer* monthly BH visits at MTFs following the onset of the pandemic compared with 2019. In contrast, there were significantly *more* monthly BH visits delivered by TRICARE-contracted private-sector providers in 2020 than in 2019. Significantly fewer BH visits were delivered by social workers and primary care providers in April–September 2020 than in 2019. The pattern of BH visits delivered in primary care and BH specialty care settings did not differ significantly between the two periods.
- **Treatment visits:** Significantly fewer group psychotherapy visits were delivered in 2020 than in 2019, but the patterns of delivery of individual psychotherapy and medication management visits did not differ significantly between the two periods.
- **Utilization after initiation of an NTE:** Cohorts of service members with an NTE for PTSD, depression, or SUD in the first three months of the study periods were *smaller* in April–September 2020 than during the same months of 2019, suggesting that fewer service members started care for these conditions in 2020. Service members who initiated treatment for PTSD or depression received significantly *more* visits in 2020 in the three months after initiating treatment. We did not observe this difference for SUD. Service members who initiated treatment for PTSD, depression, or SUD and received any individual psychotherapy received more individual therapy visits in 2020 than in 2019. We did not observe a significant difference between the two periods among those who received group psychotherapy or E&M/medication management.

The tables and figures in this chapter included 30 statistical comparisons, of which 13 were statistically significant at the $p < 0.05$ level. Some caution should be used in interpreting statistically significant results, as one significant result would be expected by chance alone.

CHAPTER FOUR

Use of Telehealth Following the Onset of the Pandemic

In this chapter, we describe the shift in the use of telehealth for BH care in April–September 2020 compared with the same months in 2019. Because there was little telehealth delivery in 2019, we describe the modalities of telehealth used by source of care (direct care versus private-sector care), care setting (primary versus specialty care), and types of treatment visits (psychotherapy, E&M), with a focus on April–September 2020. We also describe the mix of telehealth versus in-person BH care delivery within three months for service members initiating an NTE of PTSD, depression, or SUD in 2020. The box below previews the key findings presented in this chapter.

Utilization of Telehealth

As noted in Chapter Two, we categorized telehealth into one of three modalities: video (synchronous [live], interactive communication using audio and video technology), audio-only

---

Overview of Telehealth Use, April–September 2019 and April–September 2020

- Use of telehealth increased dramatically in the period April–September 2020, with most telehealth visits being coded as audio-only. In-person visits became more frequent toward the end of the observation period.
- Coding differences in telehealth data suggested a lack of standardization in categorizing modalities of telehealth visits across providers.
- Most E&M/medication management visits were coded as audio-only visits, while individual psychotherapy visits were more likely to be a mix of video and audio-only visits. Group therapy visits were few and mostly coded as delivered via video.
- Most individual psychotherapy (66 percent) and E&M/medication management visits (75 percent) were delivered via telehealth in April 2020, but these proportions dropped by September of that year (45 percent and 55 percent, respectively).

(synchronous [live], interactive communication using a telephone or other audio-only technology), and asynchronous (storing, forwarding, and transmitting of medical information in one direction at a time). Figure 4.1 shows that the pattern of BH telehealth (all modalities) and in-person visits differed significantly between 2019 and 2020. As expected, BH care was predominantly delivered in person in 2019, with only approximately 7,000 monthly telehealth visits, representing just 7.1 percent of all BH visits during that six-month period. In April–September 2020, telehealth visits for BH care totaled 291,439 (52.2 percent of BH visits). Monthly telehealth visits decreased steadily from a high of 58,629 (66.4 percent of BH visits) in April to 42,113 (41.6 percent of BH visits) in September while in-person visits increased in that period, presumably as pandemic-related restrictions eased.

Modalities of Telehealth Delivery

We examined codes used to designate the modality of telehealth delivered (e.g., Current Procedural Terminology [CPT]–code modifiers, CPT codes specific to telephone visits) in April–September 2020 and found apparent differences in coding between direct and private-sector care providers. Of the 291,439 BH telehealth visits between April and September 2020, 73.5 percent (214,081) occurred in direct care, and 26.5 percent (77,358) occurred in private-

FIGURE 4.1

Monthly In-Person Versus Telehealth BH Visits Among Service Members with PTSD, Depression, or SUD, 2019 and 2020

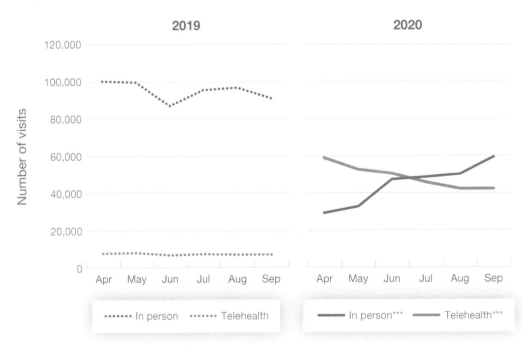

NOTES: Outpatient visits coded with a BH diagnosis in any position. *** $p < 0.001$.

sector care settings. Overall, most telehealth visits during that six-month observation period (61 percent) were coded as audio-only (results not shown). In direct care, 82.5 percent of telehealth visits were coded as audio-only, compared with only 1.1 percent of private-sector telehealth visits (Figure 4.2). In contrast, video telehealth accounted for the largest proportion of such visits in private-sector care settings, at 98.2 percent (versus 17.2 percent of direct care telehealth visits). There was minimal use of asynchronous telehealth in both direct and private-sector care settings (920 visits).

Coding of Audio-Only Telehealth

The noted variations in provider coding guidance and the large differences in observed proportions of video and audio-only telehealth between direct and private-sector care suggest variable use of codes to document telehealth modalities. Audio-only telehealth can be coded with a modifier attached to the CPT code[1] (for a service normally provided in person, such as psychotherapy or an E&M visit) or with the use of a CPT-specific code for a telehealth E&M

FIGURE 4.2

Modalities of Coded Telehealth for BH Care Among Service Members with PTSD, Depression, or SUD, by Source of Care, April–September 2020

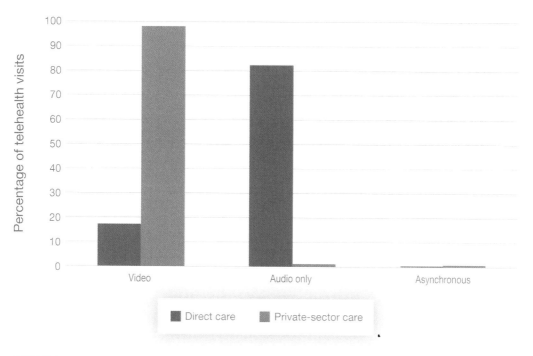

NOTE: Telehealth modality reflects coding in the administrative data.

---

[1] T2025, G2012.

visit of 5–30 minutes.[2] Of the 176,718 visits coded as audio-only visits in direct care settings, 79.5 percent were coded using audio-only CPT-code modifiers, and the remaining 21.5 percent were coded with CPT codes specific to telephone visits (telephone E&M visit lasting 5–30 minutes). In contrast, the few private-sector care telehealth visits coded as audio-only were associated with CPT telephone E&M codes. Although audio-only CPT-code modifiers were commonly used in direct care, these modifiers were not used in private-sector care (see Tables C.1 and C.2 in Appendix C).

These analyses indicated variations in how MHS providers coded telehealth visits. It is also possible that audio-only visits in private-sector care settings were coded as video telehealth, keeping with some coding guidance that defined synchronous telehealth as two-way communication with or without a visual component (Humana Military, 2020; Health Net Federal Services, undated). For these reasons, current data might preclude reliable conclusions about telehealth modality for treatment delivery.

Asynchronous Telehealth

Asynchronous telehealth represented a very small fraction (0.3 percent) of total telehealth BH care in April–September 2020, with 452 asynchronous encounters coded in direct care and 468 in private-sector care. Most asynchronous telehealth encounters in direct care involved forwarding a treatment plan to a provider or were coded as "E&M, not otherwise specified" (99499). In contrast, most asynchronous encounters in private-sector care were associated with codes for psychotherapy. It is possible that these psychotherapy visits were coded in error or based on coding guidance of which we are unaware. For example, one source of private-sector guidance for coding telehealth (not from the MHS or TRICARE) defined the modifier "GQ" as indicative of audio-only or asynchronous services (Accountable Health Partners, 2020). The noted differences in associated CPT codes and modifiers between direct care and private-sector care for asynchronous telehealth for BH care suggest some variation in coding practices and pose another potential challenge to the standardized categorization of telehealth modalities. Because of the small number of asynchronous encounters during our study periods and the potential coding issues described here, we omitted asynchronous telehealth encounters from the remaining telehealth analyses and instead focus exclusively on video and audio-only visits.

Telehealth Assessment and Treatment Visits

Figure 4.3 shows the number of psychotherapy (individual and group therapy) and BH E&M/medication management visits that were coded as delivered via telehealth in the April–September 2020 period. Individual psychotherapy telehealth visits were split fairly evenly between video (47.7 percent) and audio-only telehealth (52.3 percent). In contrast, most

---

[2] CPT codes 99441–99443 and 98966–98968.

E&M/medication management telehealth visits (79.5 percent) were coded as delivered via audio only. There were few group psychotherapy telehealth visits in this period, with most (73.6 percent) coded as conducted via video telehealth.

Proportion of Telehealth and In-Person Visits

Figure 4.4 shows the percentage of BH care visits that were delivered via telehealth in primary care versus BH specialty care settings between April and September 2020. In April 2020, 59 percent of primary care BH visits and 60 percent of BH specialty care visits were delivered via telehealth. These percentages decreased over the six-month observation period to 33 percent and 44 percent, respectively, by September. In comparison, telehealth accounted for 5.9 percent of BH primary care visits and 7.3 percent of BH specialty care visits in April 2019. These percentages remained relatively constant over the next five months of that year, with telehealth accounting for 7.0 percent and 7.3 percent of primary care and BH specialty care visits, respectively, in September 2019 (results not shown).

FIGURE 4.3

Psychotherapy and E&M/Medication Management Visits Among Service Members with PTSD, Depression, or SUD, by Modality, April–September 2020

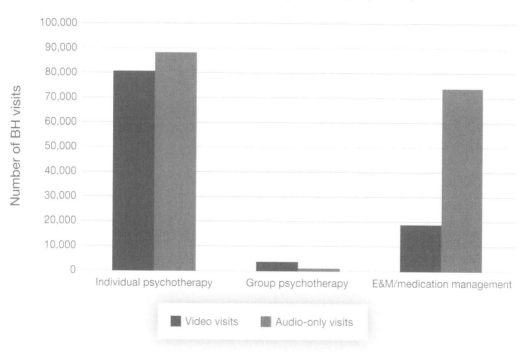

NOTES: Outpatient visits coded with a BH diagnosis in any position. Telehealth modality reflects coding in the administrative data.

FIGURE 4.4

Percentage of BH Visits Delivered via Telehealth Among Service Members with PTSD, Depression, or SUD, by Primary Care or BH Specialty Care, April–September 2020

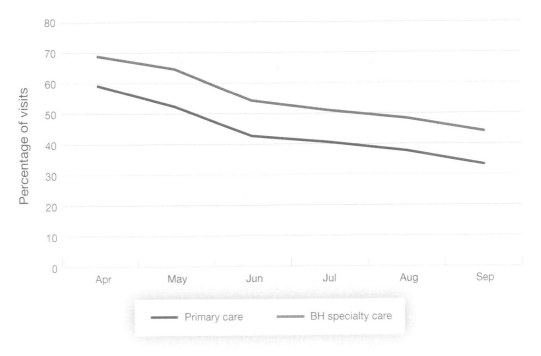

NOTE: Outpatient visits coded with a BH diagnosis in any position.

Figure 4.5 shows the percentage of treatment visits that were provided via telehealth as opposed to in person between April and September 2020. In April, 66 percent of individual psychotherapy visits and 75 percent of E&M/medication management visits were delivered via telehealth, compared with 33 percent of group therapy visits. These percentages decreased over the six-month observation period to 45 percent, 55 percent, and 24 percent, respectively, by September 2020. The proportion of treatment visits delivered via telehealth was relatively constant over the April–September 2019 period for individual psychotherapy and E&M/medication management. In September 2019, telehealth accounted for 1.2 percent of individual psychotherapy visits and 24.2 percent of E&M/medication management visits. There were no group psychotherapy visits delivered via telehealth in April–September 2019 (results not shown).

As noted in Chapter Three (Table 3.1), we identified three cohorts of service members with an NTE for PTSD, depression, or SUD who were diagnosed in the first three months (April–June) of each observation period. We examined the proportions of service members with an NTE who received BH care within three months after an initial visit via telehealth or in person between April and September 2020. Most of these service members received BH care via a combination of telehealth and in-person visits (as shown in Figure 4.6, 51.0 percent of

FIGURE 4.5

Percentage of Psychotherapy and E&M/Medication Management Visits Delivered via Telehealth Among Service Members with PTSD, Depression, or SUD, April–September 2020

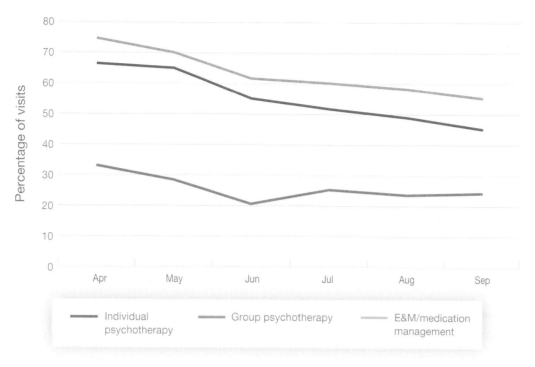

those with an NTE for PTSD, 50.5 percent with an NTE for depression, and 56.1 percent with an NTE for SUD). The corresponding shares of service members with NTEs for these conditions who received a mix of telehealth and in-person care were 17.0 percent, 21.5 percent, and 28.9 percent, respectively, in the same period in 2019 (not shown). About one-quarter of those with PTSD (25.0 percent) or depression (24.4 percent) and 13.8 percent of those with SUD received BH care only via telehealth in 2020 (Figure 4.6), compared with less than 2 percent for all conditions in 2019 (not shown).

Summary

We examined changes in the number of BH visits delivered via telehealth versus in person to service members with PTSD, depression, or SUD in April–September 2020 compared with the same months in 2019. For the studied months in 2020, we examined the use of telehealth for BH care and how these visits were coded by direct and private-sector care providers. In addition, we summarized the monthly percentage of BH visits provided via telehealth in pri-

FIGURE 4.6

Number of Service Members with a New Treatment Episode Who Received In-Person or Telehealth BH Care Within Three Months, April–September 2020

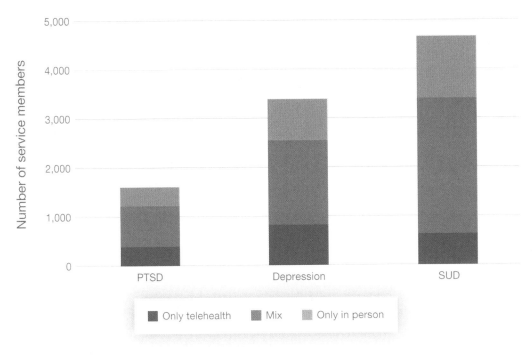

NOTE: Outpatient visits coded with a target diagnosis in any position.

mary versus BH specialty care settings and by type of visit. We also described the proportion of telehealth and in-person care delivered to service members with an NTE of PTSD, depression, or SUD. Observations from these analyses included the following:

- **Increased use of telehealth:** As expected, BH care was predominantly delivered in person in 2019; we observed only approximately 7,000 monthly telehealth visits between April and September of that year. In that same period in 2020, following the onset of the COVID-19 pandemic, monthly telehealth visits for BH care ranged from approximately 42,000 to 59,000 and totaled 291,439. Telehealth visits steadily decreased between April and September 2020, while in-person visits increased. It is unknown whether these changes were the result of easing pandemic-era restrictions or other factors. This is consistent with utilization trends in civilian data, which suggest that visit volumes in ambulatory care practices trended toward returning to baseline and that telehealth use was declining by October 2020 (Mehrotra et al., 2021).
- **Source of care:** Most direct care BH telehealth visits (83 percent) were coded as audio-only, whereas most private-sector telehealth visits (98 percent) were coded as video visits. Use of asynchronous telehealth was rare in both direct and private-sector care.

- **Coding of telehealth:** We noted differences between direct and private-sector care in the codes used to document telehealth visits. CPT modifiers for audio-only visits were common in direct care but were not used in private-sector care. Variable coding could reflect differences in provider guidance released during the observation period that did not consistently distinguish between video and audio-only visits. This variation also suggests that telehealth visits coded as video visits might have included audio-only visits.
- **Treatment visits:** Between April and September 2020, most E&M/medication management telehealth visits were coded as audio-only, while individual psychotherapy telehealth visits were an approximately equal mix of video and audio-only. The few group therapy sessions that were delivered via telehealth were coded as video visits.
- **Telehealth versus in-person care:** In April 2020, 66 percent of individual psychotherapy visits, 75 percent of E&M/medication management visits, and 33 percent of group therapy visits were delivered via telehealth. These percentages decreased over the six-month observation period to 45 percent, 55 percent, and 24 percent, respectively, by September 2020. Most service members who initiated an NTE for PTSD, depression, or SUD in April–June 2020 received a mix of in-person and telehealth BH visits in the three months after initiating care.

The tables and figures in this chapter included two statistical comparisons, of which two were statistically significant at the $p < 0.05$ level. Some caution should be used in interpreting statistically significant results because we would expect less than one significant result by chance alone.

CHAPTER FIVE

Quality of Behavioral Health Care Following the Onset of the Pandemic

In this chapter, we compare a selected set of measures reflecting aspects of the quality of BH care delivered to service members with PTSD, depression, or SUD in 2019 versus 2020 to evaluate whether there was a decrease in the quality of BH care in the MHS following the onset of the pandemic and associated physical distancing requirements. We applied 21 measures to assess various aspects of BH care quality, including whether service members received recommended care after initiating an NTE ("initial care"; seven measures), whether they received appropriate medication treatment ("medication management"; eight measures), and whether they received timely outpatient follow-up care following an inpatient discharge or ED visit ("transitions of care"; six measures).

Findings presented in Chapters Three and Four provide important context for this evaluation of the quality of BH care. In Chapter Three, we found that, overall, there were 50,000 *fewer* BH visits during the 2020 period than in the 2019 period, although the monthly pattern between the two years was not significantly different. Furthermore, we saw that service members who initiated care following the onset of the pandemic tended to receive more care compared with service members who initiated care in the pre-pandemic period. In Chapter Four, we observed a dramatic increase in the proportion of BH visits provided via telehealth in the observed months in 2020 compared with the same months in 2019.

The quality measures used in this chapter assess the delivery of recommended care (e.g., psychotherapy), regardless of the care modality (i.e., in person or via telehealth) or source (i.e., direct or private-sector care). The box below highlights key findings for this chapter.

Overview of Care Quality, April–September 2019 and April–September 2020

- BH care quality was largely sustained or improved in the period following the onset of the pandemic, with ten of 21 measures indicating similar quality and seven of 21 measures indicating improved quality in 2020 compared with 2019.
- Across both periods, receipt of recommended care was lowest on measures that assessed receipt of timely treatment or follow-up.

Measure Results: Initial Care

The seven measures addressing initial care assessed the timing and type of care received by service members who begin an NTE for PTSD, depression, or SUD. An NTE was defined as beginning with a visit for the condition after a period of no care for the condition (inpatient, outpatient, or medication). These measures assessed whether service members received any recommended treatment (e.g., psychotherapy or medication) and whether a minimally adequate number of visits was delivered in the months following the start of the NTE. Quality results for the seven measures addressing initial care are shown in Table 5.1.

Psychotherapy or Medication for New Treatment Episode

Rates of receipt of any psychotherapy or medication within four months of diagnosis for PTSD and depression were similar in April–September 2020 and the same months in 2019 (Table 5.1). Among service members with a SUD NTE, significantly fewer received any psychotherapy in April–September 2020 than in the same months in 2019. This is consistent with the analysis presented in Chapter Three, which showed lower monthly utilization for service members with SUD in 2020.

Initial Care for New Treatment Episode

Less than 40 percent of service members with an NTE for PTSD or depression received either four psychotherapy or two E&M visits in the first eight weeks after diagnosis in both 2019 and 2020, but rates were significantly *higher* in 2020 (Table 5.1). In the period prior to the pandemic (April–September 2019), most service members who received recommended care received that care *entirely* through in-person visits (82.6 percent for PTSD; 75.4 percent for depression). In the period following the onset to the pandemic, the proportion who received recommended care through telehealth markedly increased. Only about one-quarter of service members with PTSD or depression received all their recommended care via in-person visits (28.4 percent for PTSD; 24.8 percent for depression). Approximately one-third received recommended care entirely via telehealth (35.2 percent for PTSD; 36.4 percent for depression), and just over one-third received a mix of both types of care (36.3 percent for PTSD; 38.9 percent for depression).

Initiation and Engagement for AOD Care

For service members with a SUD NTE, we assessed the number who initiated care for SUD within 14 days of the new diagnosis (e.g., had at least one SUD-related visit) and the number who engaged with SUD treatment by having two or more SUD-related treatment encounters within 30 days (Table 5.1). Measure scores for initiation and engagement, while low in both periods, were significantly *higher* in the observed months in 2020 (8 percent) than in the same months in 2019 (7 percent). For 61.0 percent who engaged with treatment, the first

TABLE 5.1

Initial Care: Percentage of Service Members with a New Treatment Episode for PTSD, Depression, or SUD who Received Recommended Care, 2019 and 2020

Denominator	Numerator	April–September 2019 % (denominator)	April–September 2020 % (denominator)
Psychotherapy or medication for NTE			
Patients with a PTSD NTE	Psychotherapy or SSRI/SNRI within 4 months	76.2 (1,233)	78.8 (926)
Patients with a depression NTE	Psychotherapy or antidepressant within 4 months	75.8 (3,044)	75.5 (2,005)
Patients with an SUD NTE	Psychotherapy in 6-month observation period***	54.5 (9,947)	↓50.1 (8,259)
Initial care for NTE			
Patients with a PTSD NTE	4 psychotherapy visits or 2 E&M visits in first 8 weeks***	28.5 (2,464)	↑35.8 (2,261)
Patients with a depression NTE	4 psychotherapy visits or 2 E&M visits in first 8 weeks***	23.3 (5,799)	↑27.0 (4,571)
Initiation and engagement for AOD care			
Patients with an AOD NTE	Initiation of AOD treatment within 14 days***	18.5 (9,947)	↑22.4 (8,259)
Patients with an AOD NTE	Engagement with AOD treatment with 2 or more encounters within 30 days*	7.3 (9,947)	↑ 8.2 (8,259)

NOTES: Results include all telehealth encounters including audio-only encounters with an appropriate provider as required by the measure. Arrows denote statistically significant changes. * $p < 0.05$; *** $p < 0.001$.

engagement encounter was in person (compared with 82.9 percent in 2019), for 29.7 percent, it was via telehealth (compared with 7.9 percent in 2019), and for 8.8 percent, engagement was initiated with an inpatient stay (9.0 percent in 2019).

Measure Results: Medication Management

The eight measures that address medication management assess the duration of a newly pre-scribed medication (SSRI/SNRIs for patients with PTSD and antidepressants for patients with depression), the initiation of medication for AUD or OUD, and whether a follow-up visit occurred in the 30 days following dispensing of the newly prescribed medication. These measures reflect the importance of an adequate duration of medication treatment and timely evaluation for response to medication treatment and potential side effects. Quality results for the eight measures addressing medication management are shown in Table 5.2.

Adequate Trial of New Medication

Rates of receipt of an adequate trial of new medication for PTSD were similar in the 2019 and 2020 observation periods, whereas the proportion who received an adequate trial of a new antidepressant for depression was significantly *higher* in the April–September 2020 period compared with the same months in 2019 (Table 5.2).

Initiation of Medication for New Treatment Episode

Rates of initiating medication treatment for an NTE for AUD or OUD during the observed months in 2020 were comparable to the same period in 2019 but were low overall: 43–44 percent for AUD and 12–14 percent for OUD.

TABLE 5.2

Medication Management: Percentage of Service Members with PTSD, Depression, or SUD Who Received Recommended Care, 2019 and 2020

Denominator	Numerator	April–September 2019 % (denominator)	April–September 2020 % (denominator)
Adequate trial of new medication			
Patients with PTSD and a newly initiated SSRI/SNRI[a]	SSRI/SNRI duration ≥60 days	78.7 (1,505)	80.0 (1,142)
Patients with depression and a newly initiated antidepressant[a]	Antidepressant duration ≥12 weeks*	73.4 (3,585)	↑ 75.7 (2,733)
Initiation of medication for NTE			
Patients with an AUD NTE	Initiated AUD medication within 6-month observation period	11.5 (8,980)	12.3 (7,458)
Patients with an OUD NTE	Initiated OUD medication within 6-month observation period	13.9 (1,519)	12.7 (1,018)
Follow-up visit after new medication			
Patients with PTSD and newly initiated SSRI/SNRI	E&M visit within 30 days**	43.7 (2,500)	↓ 39.5 (2,305)
Patients with depression and newly initiated antidepressant	E&M visit within 30 days**	42.0 (7,024)	↓ 39.5 (6,315)
Patients with AUD and newly initiated AUD medication	E&M visit within 30 days	43.6 (1,032)	43.2 (914)
Patients with OUD and newly initiated OUD medication	E&M visit within 30 days	14.2 (211)	11.6 (129)

NOTES: Results include all telehealth encounters including telephone-only encounters with an appropriate provider as required by the measure. Arrows denote statistically significant changes. * $p < 0.05$; ** $p < 0.01$.

[a] Required a condition diagnosis in the 60 days prior to or after new medication dispensing.

Follow-Up Visit After New Medication

The proportion of service members who received a follow-up visit within 30 days after initiating a new medication for PTSD or depression was significantly *lower* during the observed six months in 2020 than during the same months in 2019. Rates of follow-up following initiation of medication for AUD or OUD were similar during both periods, but scores were low, particularly for OUD. Among those who received a timely follow-up visit in April–September 2020, the first follow-up was a telehealth visit for 63.7 percent for PTSD, 57.6 percent for depression, 67.3 percent for AUD, and 73.3 percent for OUD. In April–September 2019, corresponding first follow-up visits via telehealth were 17.9 percent, 15.8 percent, 36.4 percent, and 30 percent, respectively.

Measure Results: Transitions of Care

The six quality measures related to transitions of care address follow-up after discharge from inpatient or ED settings and included discharges from both direct and private-sector care facilities. These measures focus on the vulnerable period during transitions of care when patient conditions and treatment plans may have changed and continuing care is vital to providing appropriate ongoing treatment. Quality measure results for the six measures addressing transitions of care are shown in Table 5.3.

TABLE 5.3

Transitions of Care: Percentage of Discharges Among Service Members with PTSD, Depression, or SUD with Recommended Care, 2019 and 2020

Denominator	Numerator	April–September 2019 (%, denominator)	April–September 2020 (%, denominator)
Follow-up after psychiatric hospitalization			
Psychiatric hospitalization discharges	Follow-up within 7 days[a]	80.9 (4,955)	79.8 (3,977)
Psychiatric hospitalization discharges	Follow-up within 30 days[a]**	91.9 (4,955)	↓90.0 (3,977)
Follow-up after ED visit for MH or AOD			
MH-related ED visits	Follow-up within 7 days	53.3 (1,980)	54.2 (1,576)
MH-related ED visits	Follow-up within 30 days	68.8 (1,980)	69.2 (1,576)
AOD-related ED visits	Follow-up within 7 days**	16.9 (884)	↑ 23.3 (622)
AOD-related ED visits	Follow-up within 30 days***	25.6 (884)	↑ 35.0 (622)

NOTES: Results include all telehealth encounters, including telephone-only encounters with an appropriate provider as required by the measure. Arrows denote statistically significant changes. ** $p < 0.01$; *** $p < 0.001$.

[a] Numerator does not include follow-up visits on the day of hospital discharge.

Follow-Up After Psychiatric Hospitalization

Table 5.3 shows the percentage of psychiatric inpatient discharges and MH- or AOD-related ED visits that were associated with recommended follow-up. Rates of receipt of follow-up care after inpatient psychiatric hospitalization in April–September 2020 were high overall: 80 percent and 90 percent for follow-up within seven and 30 days, respectively. While still high at 90 percent, the score for follow-up within 30 days was significantly *lower* than that in the same months of 2019. For inpatient discharges with follow-up within 30 days in April–September 2020, 96.0 percent occurred within two weeks of discharge. For inpatient discharges in the April–September 2020 observation period with a follow-up visit within seven days, 43.5 percent of first visits occurred via telehealth; for follow-up visits within 30 days, 46 percent of first visits occurred via telehealth. In contrast, first follow-up via telehealth in the April–September 2019 observation period was 15.2 percent and 16.9 percent, respectively.

Follow-Up After an ED Visit for MH or AOD

Rates of receipt of follow-up after an MH-related ED visit were similar during both observation periods. Of all the follow-up visits that occurred within 30 days in April–September 2020, 89.4 percent occurred within the first two weeks after discharge. For MH-related ED visits with follow-up, 39.2 percent of follow-up visits within seven days were delivered via telehealth in that same period, as were 43.3 percent of follow-up visits within 30 days. In comparison, these rates were 10.0 percent and 9.5 percent for telehealth follow-up within seven and 30 days, respectively, in April–September 2019.

Rates of receipt of follow-up after an AOD-related ED visit, while low, were significantly *higher* in the six-month observation period in 2020 than in the same months in 2019. Of all the follow-up visits that occurred within 30 days in the April–September 2020 observation period, 80.3 percent occurred within the first two weeks. For those with a follow-up visit within seven days or 30 days, 40.0 percent and 46.3 percent of first follow-up visits, respectively, were delivered via telehealth in April–September 2020. In comparison, these rates were 21.5 percent and 14.2 percent for telehealth follow-up within seven and 30 days, respectively, in April–September 2019.

Summary

In this chapter, we compared quality of BH care for service members with PTSD, depression, or SUD in two six-month periods (April–September 2019 and April–September 2020). Denominators for all measures—the number of eligible service members or discharges—were lower in 2020 than in 2019, reflecting that fewer service members were seen for these conditions in 2020. In comparing BH care quality in the two periods, results were mixed but suggested that the quality of BH care was largely maintained following the onset of the pandemic. Of the 21 measures, nearly half did not differ significantly between the 2019 and 2020 periods (ten measures). For seven measures, scores were significantly *higher* in 2020. In contrast, scores were significantly *lower* for four measures. The quality measures with the lowest rates of delivery of recommended care involved service members' receipt of recommended care related to timely delivery of an adequate amount of treatment for an NTE and follow-up after initiation of new medication, findings that were similar to those from a prior study (Hepner, Brown, et al., 2021). Table 5.4 provides an overview of the measure results presented in this chapter.

As shown in Chapter Four, a much larger proportion of BH care was delivered via telehealth in April–September 2020 than in the same period in 2019. Our analyses of BH care quality did not compare the quality of care by mode of delivery (i.e., in person versus telehealth). Thus, we can only infer the potential impact of telehealth from our comparison of one period with very little telehealth (2019) and one with a substantial amount of telehealth (2020). Thus, it is notable that the quality of BH care was largely sustained—and even improved in some respects—in the context of pandemic-related restrictions and the expanded use of telehealth. Our analyses allowed both video and audio-only coded telehealth visits (with an appropriate provider) to qualify as follow-up visits. Our supplementary analyses found that the inclusion of specific telephone E&M codes (visits 5–30 minutes in duration with a qualifying provider) increased the rates of follow-up scores for some measures by a small percentage (see Table D.1 in Appendix D).

Key findings were as follows:

- **Initial care:** Scores on six of seven measures assessing receipt of recommended initial care were similar or improved in 2020 compared with 2019. Similar proportions of service members with an NTE for PTSD or depression received any recommended treatment (psychotherapy or medication) in 2020 and 2019. However, significantly *fewer* service members who started treatment for SUD received any psychotherapy in 2020 than in 2019. Significantly *more* service members initiating care for PTSD or depression received at least a minimal amount of recommended care in 2020 than in 2019. Similarly, significantly *more* service members with SUD received at least minimal visits. Scores on these measures in 2020 varied widely—from 8 percent to 79 percent—suggesting several areas for improvement.

TABLE 5.4

Quality Measure Score Changes from 2019 to 2020

Measure Domain (number of measures)	April–September 2020 Scores versus April–September 2019 (number of measures)			April–September 2020 Scores (number of measures)	
	Lower	Same	Higher	Score ≥50	Score ≥75
Initial care (7)	1	2	4	3	2
Medication management (8)	2	5	1	2	2
Transitions of care (6)	1	3	2	4	2
Total	4	10	7	9	6

- **Medication management**: Scores on six of eight measures assessing receipt of recommended medication treatment were similar or improved in 2020 compared with 2019. Service members who initiated medication treatment for depression in 2020 were significantly more likely to receive an adequate duration of medication; rates were similar for PTSD. Rates for initiation of medication for service members initiating treatment for AUD or OUD were similar between the time periods. Receipt of follow-up after initiation of new medication was significantly lower in April–September 2020 than in the same months in 2019 for PTSD and depression (40 percent for both PTSD and depression in 2020 versus 44 percent and 42 percent in 2019, respectively). Rates of timely follow-up after initiation of new medication were mixed, with two measures showing similar rates (for AUD and OUD) and two measures indicating significantly *worse* rates of follow-up (for PTSD and depression). Scores on these measures in 2020 varied widely—from 12 percent to 80 percent—suggesting several areas for improvement.
- **Transitions of care:** Scores on five of six measures assessing receipt of timely outpatient follow-up after an MH inpatient or ED discharge were similar or improved in 2020 compared with 2019. During both periods, timely follow-up after inpatient care was high, but follow-up was generally lower after ED visits. Although still high, the rate of timely outpatient follow-up within 30 days was significantly lower than in 2019. The rate was not significantly different for seven-day follow-up. Scores for follow-up after MH-related ED visits were similar in both periods. Scores for AOD-related ED visit follow-up, while low, were significantly higher in 2020 than in 2019. Scores on these measures in 2020 varied widely—from 23 percent to 90 percent—suggesting several areas for improvement.

The tables and figures in this chapter include 21 statistical comparisons, of which 11 were statistically significant at the $p < 0.05$ level. Some caution should be used in interpreting statistically significant results, as one significant result would be expected by chance alone.

CHAPTER SIX

Key Findings and Recommendations

In this report, we examined changes in BH care delivery following the onset of the COVID-19 pandemic, including BH care utilization patterns, use of telehealth, and the quality of BH care provided to service members with PTSD, depression, or SUD. To characterize changes in patterns of care, we compared two six-month periods: April–September 2019, prior to the onset of the pandemic, and April–September 2020, after pandemic-related restrictions on care delivery were implemented. This chapter highlights the strengths and limitations of the analyses, presents key findings, and offers policy recommendations and directions for future research.

Strengths and Limitations

The analyses presented in this report have several strengths. First, the administrative data we used in our analyses were comprehensive: They included both direct care (delivered at MTFs) and private-sector care (delivered by TRICARE-contracted providers). Thus, we analyzed all coded BH care paid for by the MHS for active-component service members with a diagnosis of PTSD, depression, or SUD in April–September 2019 and April–September 2020. Second, to mitigate the effects of seasonal variation in health care utilization on our analysis, we compared care delivered in two parallel six-month periods. The 2020 period provided an opportunity to observe care utilization trends beginning soon after the implementation of pandemic-related restrictions on in-person care delivery (April 2020) through a time when in-person care was increasing (September 2020). Finally, we applied a broad range of administrative data–based quality measures to assess the quality of care for PTSD, depression, and SUD delivered during the two periods.

The analyses in this report also have some limitations. First, we presented preliminary descriptive analyses of outpatient BH care utilization within selected date ranges for three target BH diagnoses. We supplemented our descriptive analyses with statistical modeling that compared patterns of care between the two periods. These regression models did not control for patient characteristics or other factors that could affect the comparability of the two periods. Second, the administrative data used in our analyses reflect patterns of utilization and do not capture potential changes in the need for BH care or patient preferences regarding telehealth. Civilian data suggest that BH care needs may have increased after the onset of the COVID-19 pandemic (McGinty et al., 2020; Ettman et al., 2020). Third, fewer patients with PTSD, depression, or SUD were seen during the 2020 period relative to 2019, which may have implications for the interpretation of our findings, particularly with respect to the quality of BH care delivered. Fourth, MHS and TRICARE definitions of telehealth modalities and coding guidance for video and audio-only telehealth visits were not consistent. There was likely provider- and clinic-level variability in the way telehealth codes were used, which may further limit the generalizability of our findings—particularly with respect to video versus audio-only telehealth. Finally, although we were able analyze the quality of BH care in several domains, administrative data–based quality measures cannot capture certain details about the care delivered, such as whether psychotherapy was evidence-based, the quality of the patient-provider interaction, and appropriate uses of telehealth. We also were unable to assess whether service member BH outcomes changed between the two periods because of limitations on outcome monitoring during the pandemic. As discussed in a recent RAND report (Hepner, Sousa, et al., 2021), MHS providers typically use the BHDP to track symptom assessment data collected from patients through tablets or waiting room kiosks, something that was not feasible during the pandemic. Particularly with the widespread, increased use of telehealth following the onset of the pandemic, there is a need to understand whether BH outcomes were sustained during 2020 and beyond.

Despite these limitations, this report offers a preliminary assessment of BH care utilization patterns, use of telehealth, and quality of care for active-component service members with PTSD, depression, or SUD during the period following the onset of the COVID-19 pandemic.

Key Findings

In this section, we provide an overview of key findings from our analyses.

Pandemic-Related Restrictions Prompted Changes in Behavioral Health Care Delivery

We observed several differences between April–September 2019 and April–September 2020 in terms of monthly BH care utilization by BH diagnosis, treatment type, provider type, and source of care. Overall, there were 50,000 fewer BH visits during the 2020 period than in the 2019 period, although the monthly pattern between the two years was not significantly different. The pattern of monthly BH care utilization for SUD, specifically, was significantly different between the two periods, indicating *fewer* visits for SUD in the 2020 pandemic period than in 2019; patterns did not differ for PTSD or depression. Furthermore, there were significantly *fewer* group psychotherapy visits in the 2020 pandemic period than in the 2019 period, but the pattern did not differ for individual therapy or medication management visits. The decrease in group therapy is consistent with findings of from previous RAND research suggesting that many military providers found group psychotherapy challenging to deliver via telehealth, with many electing to suspend sessions to support physical distancing (Hepner, Sousa, et al., 2021).

We also identified diverging patterns in direct versus private-sector care settings. In direct care settings (i.e., at MTFs), where the majority of BH visits occurred for active-component service members with PTSD, depression, or SUD, there were significantly *fewer* monthly BH visits in the 2020 pandemic period than in 2019. The opposite was true in private-sector care settings (i.e., where care is delivered by TRICARE-contracted providers): There were significantly *more* monthly BH visits in the 2020 pandemic period than in 2019. Hepner and colleagues (Hepner, Sousa, et al., 2021) reported that BH care at some MTFs was halted for several months during the pandemic, and the volume of care significantly decreased in others. Clinic closures and challenges associated with rapid telehealth implementation could have affected utilization patterns differently in direct and private-sector care settings. We found that there were significantly fewer BH visits delivered by primary care providers and social workers during the 2020 pandemic period than in 2019, but we did not detect a difference for other BH providers.

There were also significant differences in the BH care received by service members with an NTE. Fewer service members initiated treatment for PTSD, depression, and SUD in April–September 2020 than in April–September 2019. It is unclear whether this difference was a result of limited access to appointments or a reduced need for care. Notably, the service members who initiated care for PTSD or depression in 2020 had significantly *more* visits within the first three months than service members with an NTE for PTSD or depression in 2019. Service members with an NTE in 2020 for PTSD, depression, or SUD who received individual psychotherapy also had *more* individual psychotherapy visits than their counterparts in 2019.

Telehealth Use Increased Markedly After the Onset of the Pandemic but Varied by Type of Treatment

The pattern of BH telehealth and in-person visits differed significantly between 2019 and 2020. As expected, BH care in the MHS was delivered primarily in person in April–September 2019, a period that saw only approximately 7,000 monthly telehealth visits. During the same period in 2020, there were approximately 42,000–59,000 visits monthly telehealth visits for BH care. Most of the telehealth visits during this time (61 percent) were coded as audio-only. The highest monthly volume of telehealth occurred in April 2020, when 66 percent of individual psychotherapy and 75 percent of E&M/medication management visits were provided via telehealth. Between April and September 2020, telehealth visits steadily decreased while in-person visits increased, presumably as pandemic-restrictions eased.

Patterns of telehealth use varied by type of treatment. In April–September 2020, most E&M/medication management telehealth visits were coded as audio-only, while individual psychotherapy telehealth visits were an approximately equal mix of video and audio-only modalities. Few group therapy visits were coded as having been delivered via telehealth, and most of those were coded as video visits. Most service members initiating an NTE for PTSD, depression, or SUD in April–June 2020 received a mix of in-person and telehealth BH visits in the three months after initiating care. Telehealth modalities also varied between direct and private-sector care settings. Most direct care telehealth visits (83 percent) were coded as audio-only, while most private-sector telehealth visits (98 percent) were coded as video visits. It is difficult to accurately assess the use of video versus audio-only care because of variability in provider guidance regarding definitions of telehealth modalities and related coding.

Behavioral Health Care Quality Was Largely Sustained or Improved Following the Onset of the Pandemic, Although Fewer Service Members Were Seen for PTSD, Depression, or SUD

We used 21 measures to evaluate the quality of BH care provided to service members in the April–September 2019 and 2020 periods. These measures addressed the domains of initial care, medication management, and transitions of care. The quality of BH care was largely sustained or improved in the period following the onset of the pandemic, with ten of 21 measures showing similar care quality and seven measures showing improvement in April–September 2020 compared with 2019. Although fewer service members with PTSD, depression, or SUD were seen in 2020, our data indicated that the MHS was able to provide them with care of comparable quality to what they would have received in 2019, despite the challenges imposed by the pandemic.

Six of seven measure scores addressing initial care held steady or improved between 2019 and 2020. Fewer service members with a new SUD diagnosis received any psychotherapy, but more service members with an NTE of PTSD, depression, or SUD received a minimal amount of recommended care. Scores for six of eight measures addressing medication management were similar or improved. More service members with depression and a new antidepressant received an adequate trial of medication. However, fewer service members with PTSD or depression who initiated new medication treatment received a follow-up visit within 30 days. Scores on five of six measures of timely outpatient follow-up after transitions of care were similar or improved. Scores for follow-up after psychiatric hospitalization within 30 days were lower in 2020 than in 2019, but more AOD-related ED visits were associated with follow-up visits within seven or 30 days than in 2019. Scores in each domain of care varied widely from 8 percent to 90 percent, suggesting several areas for improvement. Receipt of recommended care was lowest in both years when it came to the timely delivery of treatment or follow-up.

Policy Implications

Recommendation 1. Continue the Expanded Use of Telehealth for Behavioral Health Care and Monitor Care Quality

Our analyses highlighted a marked expansion in the use of telehealth following the onset of pandemic-related restrictions. Although the MHS was already taking steps to integrate telehealth into BH care delivery (U.S. House of Representatives, 2016; Pamplin et al., 2019), the pandemic required a rapid, evolving response to ensure care availability and continuity (Mehrotra et al., 2020; MHS Communications Office, 2020; Uscher-Pines et al., 2020). The MHS went from approximately 7,000 monthly telebehavioral health visits in April–September 2019 to approximately 42,000–59,000 visits per month in the same period in 2020—with the highest number of telehealth visits in April 2020. Despite this rapid, evolving transition, our analyses suggest that the overall quality of BH care did not decline in 2020. In fact, we observed that the rates at which service members received recommended care for PTSD, depression, and SUD were sustained (ten of 21 measures) or improved (seven measures) between 2019 and 2020. One important caveat in interpreting these findings is that fewer service members with these conditions were treated following the onset of the pandemic. This could have been because service members delayed care or because of a lack of available appointments (Jowers, 2020). Still, these findings provide promising support for the ongoing widespread use of telehealth as part of BH care delivery in the MHS.

We recommend that the MHS continue to expand its use of telehealth, alongside efforts to monitor BH care quality on an ongoing basis, rather than reducing telehealth delivery to pre-pandemic levels. Our 2020 data showed gradual decreases in telehealth and increases in in-person care over time, suggesting the possibility of a gradual return to pre-pandemic operations. This is consistent with utilization trends in civilian data, which suggest that visit volumes in ambulatory care practices were trending toward returning to baseline and telehealth use was declining by October 2020 (Mehrotra et al., 2021). A RAND study of military BH providers' perspectives on telehealth following the onset of the pandemic recommended that the MHS develop policy guidance on the use of telehealth for patients with specific BH conditions, develop and implement a strategic plan to ensure that providers have adequate technology to support video telehealth, and provide clinical and technical training on the use of telehealth (Hepner, Sousa, et al., 2021). These continue to be important steps to support ongoing telehealth implementation. This report provides additional insights for these efforts. It will be important to continue monitoring BH care access and quality to ensure that they are sustained with the use of telehealth. Our analyses of BH care quality identified strengths and ongoing areas for improvement for the MHS.

Telehealth will likely play an important role in preparedness for future disruptions in care, from pandemics to natural disasters; for this reason, it should be integrated into future planning (Alverson et al., 2010; Lurie and Carr, 2018; Smith et al., 2020). We note that it appears that BH visits delivered by military providers *decreased* following the onset of the pandemic, while BH visits delivered by private-sector providers *increased* during this same period. It is important to gain a better understanding of the mechanisms underlying these changing patterns of care. This also raises questions about whether the MHS could better prepare MTFs for future potential disruptions in care and how telehealth could support the MHS's ability to rapidly adapt when needed.

Recommendation 2. Assess Behavioral Health Treatment Outcomes Among Service Members Who Receive Telehealth

Our analyses were limited to evaluating process measures related to the quality of BH care delivered to service members with PTSD, depression, or SUD. These analyses suggest that BH care quality in most areas of care studied did not decrease with the marked expansion of telehealth following the pandemic's onset, although there is reason for caution in interpreting this finding because we also found that fewer service members were seen. We were not able to compare treatment outcomes (e.g., symptom improvement) between the 2019 and 2020 periods because pandemic-related restrictions limited data collection in 2020. Prior to the pandemic, routine collection of patient symptoms relied on BHDP waiting room kiosks and tablets—data collection methods that were not feasible for telehealth visits. Although some BH providers collected the data orally during the session, most temporarily stopped collecting patient symptom measures (Hepner, Sousa, et al., 2021). The MHS is planning to expand BHDP capabilities to allow patient-reported measures to be collected remotely, increasing the feasibility of collecting these data prior to telehealth visits. This will be an important step in accurately tracking symptoms across modes of care delivery and providing essential data to compare outcomes for patients who receive telehealth. Existing research suggests that BH outcomes are comparable between in-person and telehealth delivery for numerous conditions (Backhaus et al., 2012; Bashshur et al., 2014; Fortney et al., 2015; Gentry et al., 2019; Hilty et al., 2013; Rosen et al., 2021). In fact, BH applications of telehealth are among the most widely studied, relative to other specialties (Baer, Elford, and Cukor, 1997; Shigekawa et al., 2018). However, telehealth has historically been underutilized in SUD treatment, and more research may be needed to confirm long-term BH treatment effects with its use (Lin, Fernandez, and Bonar, 2020; Olthuis et al., 2016). Furthermore, it is important to demonstrate that treatment outcomes, such as symptom reduction, are comparable between in-person and telehealth modalities (i.e., video, audio-only). It would also be valuable to assess service members' perceptions of their experiences with BH care and their views on the advantages and disadvantages of telehealth.

Recommendation 3. Increase the Clarity of Telehealth Coding Guidance for Providers

Our review of the provider guidance for telehealth coding provided by the MHS and TRICARE at the start of the pandemic revealed some variation in the definitional categories of telehealth modalities. *Synchronous telehealth* was defined as video visits in some documentation (MHS, 2020; DHA, 2020; National Capital Consortium Pediatrics, 2020), but, elsewhere, it was described more broadly as two-way communication in a way that did not distinguish between video and audio-only visits (Health Net Federal Services, undated; Humana Military, 2020). Our analyses of BH care delivered via telehealth in April–September 2020 revealed marked differences in the telehealth modalities coded by direct care and private-sector care providers. Most telehealth during the 2020 observation period (74 percent) was delivered by direct care providers, and most of these visits (83 percent) were coded as audio-only. In contrast, almost all private-sector care telehealth visits (98 percent) were coded as (synchronous) video visits. MHS and TRICARE guidance that did not consistently distinguish between video and audio-only visits meant that it was unclear whether these private-sector care visits included audio-only visits, and, if they did, what proportion of these visits were video versus audio-only. It is understandable that provider guidance was evolving during the early months of the pandemic in response to a rapidly changing situation. Whether or not the MHS continues to expand its use of telehealth, we recommend that providers across direct and private-sector care settings receive coding guidance with standardized definitions of telehealth modalities and associated coding for telehealth visits. Going forward, it will also be important to monitor quality and outcomes of telehealth visits. To this end, being able to reliably distinguish video visits from audio-only visits will help determine whether telehealth modality influences the quality of care, provider-patient interactions, and patient outcomes.

Conclusions

The pandemic provided a lesson in resilience for the health care sector. The MHS was already exploring options to expand telehealth integration, and our preliminary analyses support these efforts and provide insights to inform decisions about further telehealth adoption. If implemented appropriately, telehealth likely has an important role to play in strengthening military readiness and improving access to high-quality BH care for service members.

Telehealth Coding

This appendix provides details on the sources of information that guided our telehealth analyses. It includes military guidance for providers for telehealth coding that was issued early in the pandemic (Table A.1). It also includes the algorithm that we used to categorize telehealth visits (Table A.2), along with related telehealth encounter CPT codes and modifiers (Table A.3).

TABLE A.1

Military Telehealth Coding Guidance

Source	Coding	Comment
"Frequently Asked Questions: COVID-19 and Virtual Health for Providers" (MHS, 2020)	**Audio and visual encounters:** E&M service code AND [GT modifier (MTF to MTF) OR 95 modifier (provider to patient location other than MTF)] **Telephone-only encounters:** E&M service code AND T2025 (waiver services, not otherwise specified)	Current as of June 1, 2020
"Interim Virtual Encounter Guidance During COVID-19 National Emergency," attachment 3c (DHA, 2020)	**Synchronous visual and audio telecommunications:** Procedure code AND E&M code or 99499 or leave blank AND [GT modifier (MTF to MTF) OR 95 modifier (provider to patient location other than MTF)] **Telephone only:** G2012 AND E&M code 99499 or leave blank	Dated March 18, 2020 Audio and visual source is National Capital Consortium Pediatric Residency, Walter Reed National Military Medical Center

Table A.1—Continued

Source	Coding	Comment
"Telemedicine Cheat Sheet" DHA resource (National Capital Consortium Pediatrics, 2020)	**Audio/visual face-to-face encounters (Adobe Connect):** ICD10-diagnosis code AND E&M-office visit code AND Modifier- 95 or GT **95 =** synchronous audio/visual virtual encounter, patient is somewhere other than MTF (home or other appropriate setting). **GT =** synchronous audio/visual virtual encounter when the patient is at another MTF **GQ =** asynchronous virtual encounter, consulting provider is reviewing stored documentation to provide interpretation/opinion to requesting provider	Dated April 22, 2020 Audio/visual Source is National Capital Consortium Pediatrics, residency Walter Reed
	Telephone consultation coding criteria (i.e., virtual encounter, SPEC-HC): ICD-10 code for the encounter AND E&M- 99499 (unlisted E&M) AND HCPCS-T2025 code	For established patients. Does not include Nurse Advice Line
"Telemedicine Billing Tips," TRICARE West resource (Health Net Federal Services, undated)	**Synchronous telemedicine services (two directions):** CPT/HCPCS code AND [GT or 95 modifier (distant site) OR Q3014 (applicable originating site)]	Undated *Synchronous* defined as interactive electronic information exchange in at least two directions in the same period. Does not specify audio or visual
	Asynchronous telemedicine services (one direction): CPT/HCPCS code AND GQ modifier	*Asynchronous* defined as storing, forwarding, and transmitting information in one direction at a time.
	Audio-only visits: CPT 99441–43, 98966–68 and HCPCS code G2012	

Table A.1—Continued

Source	Coding	Comment
"Coronavirus Disease (COVID-19) and TRICARE's Telemedicine Benefit" (Humana Military, 2020)	**Synchronous (two directions):** CPT or HCPCS code AND GT modifier for distant site and Q3014 for an applicable originating site. Place of Service "POS 02" is to be reported in conjunction with the GT modifier	Updated April 29, 2020 *Synchronous* defined as interactive electronic information exchange in at least two directions in the same period. Does not specify audio and visual.
	Asynchronous (one direction): CPT or HCPCS codes AND GQ modifier	*Asynchronous* defined as storing, forwarding, and transmitting information in one direction at a time.

NOTES: Bold text reflects language used in the guidance document. HCPCS = Healthcare Common Procedure Coding System.

We applied the following algorithm hierarchically to categorize telehealth modalities for direct care and private-sector care visits.

TABLE A.2
Telehealth Coding Algorithm

Direct Care	Private-Sector Care
Requirements for inclusion	
CAPER/GENESIS BH visit with provider HIPAA taxonomy code associated with	TRICARE Encounter Data–Noninstitutional BH visit with provider HIPAA taxonomy code associated with
CAPER skill level 1 or 2 OR CAPER skill level 4 counselor: Counselor, counselor: addiction; counselor: mental health; counselor: professional	CAPER skill level 1 or 2 OR CAPER skill level 4 counselor: Counselor, counselor: addiction; counselor: mental health; counselor: professional
Exclusions	
• Originating procedure code Q3014[a] • Visit with technical procedure • Provider-to-provider consultation	• Originating procedure code Q3014[a] • Visit with technical procedure • Provider-to-provider consultation • PPS product line = 3 (facility)
Hierarchical categorization of telehealth visits	
Video/synchronous: [Modifier GT or 95 AND No telephone-only procedure code] OR [MEPRS = BFDR AND DMIS ID = 0047 or 0052 or 0109 (telehealth hub)]	**Video/synchronous:** [Modifier GT or 95 OR Place of service (POS) = 2] AND No telephone-only procedure code

Table A.2—Continued

Direct Care	Private-Sector Care
Asynchronous:	**Asynchronous:**
Not synchronous AND No telephone-only procedure code AND [Modifier GQ OR Asynchronous procedure code]	Same as direct care
Audio only/telephone only:	**Audio only/telephone only:**
Not synchronous AND Not asynchronous AND Telephone-only procedure code	Same as direct care

NOTES: A BH encounter is an encounter with an ICD-10 F-code. We did not include the modifier GO because it did not occur in our data. The analysis included the following coded definitions:

- HIPAA taxonomy, counselor: 101Y00000X, 101YA0400X, 101YM0800X, 101YP2500X. These counselor codes with skill level 4 were included because of our focus on BH care and the observed frequency in our data of this type of provider's being associated with encounters with a psychotherapy CPT code.
- Technical procedure: 95700, 95705–95716.
- Provider-to-provider consultation: 99446–99452.
- Telephone-only procedure: 99441–99143, 98966–98968, T2025, G2012.
- Asynchronous procedure: 92227, 92228, 93264, 95717-95726, 99453, 99454, 99457, 99458, D9996, G9868–G9870, G0071, G2010.

a Code excluded to avoid double counting of encounters.

TABLE A.3

Algorithm Telehealth Codes and Online Encounter Codes

Modifier/ CPT Code/ HCPCS Code	Description
Video/synchronous	
GT modifier	Telehealth encounter, synchronous
95 modifier	Telehealth encounter, synchronous
Asynchronous	
GQ modifier	Telehealth encounter, asynchronous
G2010	Remote evaluation of recorded video and/or images submitted by an established patient (e.g., store and forward), including interpretation with follow-up with the patient within 24 business hours, not originating from a related E&M service provided within the previous 7 days nor leading to an E&M service or procedure within the next 24 hours or soonest available appointment
92227	Remote imaging for the detection of retinal disease with analysis and report under physician supervision, unilateral or bilateral

Table A.3—Continued

Modifier/ CPT Code/ HCPCS Code	Description
92228	Remote imaging for monitoring and management of active retinal disease with physician review, interpretation, and report, unilateral or bilateral
93264	Remote monitoring of a wireless pulmonary artery pressure sensor for up to 30 days, including at least weekly downloads of pulmonary artery pressure recordings, interpretation(s), trend analysis, and report(s) by a physician or other qualified health care professional
95717	EEG, continuous recording, physician or other qualified health care professional review of recorded events, interpretation and report, 2–12 hours, without video
95718	With video
95719	EEG, continuous recording, physician or other qualified health care professional review of recorded events, analysis of spike and seizure detection, each increment of greater than 12 hours, up to 26 hours of EEG recording, interpretation and report after each 24-hour period; without video
95720	With video
95721	EEG, continuous recording, physician or other qualified health care professional review of recorded events, analysis of spike and seizure detection, interpretation, and summary report, complete study; greater than 36 hours, up to 60 hours of EEG recording, without video
95722	Greater than 36 hours, up to 60 hours of EEG recording, with video
95723	Greater than 60 hours, up to 84 hours of EEG recording, without video
95724	Greater than 60 hours, up to 84 hours of EEG recording, with video
95725	Greater than 84 hours of EEG recording, without video
95726	Greater than 84 hours of EEG recording, with video
99453	Remote monitoring of physiologic parameter(s) (e.g., weight, blood pressure, pulse oximetry, respiratory flow rate), initial; set-up and patient education on use of equipment
99454	Remote monitoring of physiologic parameter(s) (e.g., weight, blood pressure, pulse oximetry, respiratory flow rate), initial; each 30 days
99457	Remote physiologic monitoring treatment management services, 20 minutes or more of clinical staff/physician/other qualified health care professional time in a calendar month requiring interactive communication with the patient/caregiver during the month
99458	Additional 20 minutes
D9996	Asynchronous information stored and forwarded to dentist for subsequent review
G9868	Receipt and analysis of remote, asynchronous images for dermatologic and/or ophthalmologic evaluation, less than 10 minutes
G9869	10–20 minutes
G9870	More than 20 minutes

Table A.3—Continued

Modifier/ CPT Code/ HCPCS Code	Description
G0071	Communication technology-based services for 5 minutes or more of a virtual (non–face-to-face) communication between a rural health clinic or federally qualified health center practitioner and patient or 5 minutes or more of remote evaluation of recorded video and/or images by a qualified practitioner, occurring in lieu of an office visit
Audio only/telephone	
99441	Telephone evaluation and management, physician, or qualified health care professional, established patient, 5–10 minutes
99442	11–20 minutes
99443	21–30 minutes
98966	Telephone assessment and management service provided by a qualified non-physician health care professional to an established patient, 5–10 minutes
98967	11–20 minutes
98968	21–30 minutes
G2012	Brief communication technology-based service, e.g., virtual check-in, by a physician or other qualified health care professional who can report evaluation and management services, provided to an established patient, not originating from a related E&M service provided within the previous 7 days nor leading to an E&M service or procedure within the next 24 hours or soonest available appointment: 5–10 minutes
T2025	Waiver services, not otherwise specified
Exclusions	
95700	EEG continuous recording, with video when performed, setup, patient education, and takedown, administered in person by EEG technologist, minimum of 8 channels
95705	EEG without video, review of data, technical description by EEG technologist, 2–12 hours, unmonitored
95706	With intermittent monitoring and maintenance
95707	With continuous monitoring
95708	EEG without video, review of data, technical description by EEG technologist, 12–26 hours, unmonitored
95709	With intermittent monitoring and maintenance
95710	With continuous monitoring
95711	EEG with video, review of data, technical description by EEG technologist, 2–12 hours, unmonitored
95712	With intermittent monitoring and maintenance
95713	With continuous monitoring
95714	EEG with video, review of data, technical description by EEG technologist, 12–26 hours, unmonitored
95715	With intermittent monitoring and maintenance
95716	With continuous monitoring

Table A.3—Continued

Modifier/ CPT Code/ HCPCS Code	Description
99446	Interprofessional telephone/internet/electronic assessment and management service provided by a consultative physician including verbal and written report to requesting physician or other qualified health care professional, 5-10 minutes
99447	11–20 minutes
99448	21–30 minutes
99449	More than 30 minutes
99451	Interprofessional telephone/internet/electronic assessment and management service provided by a consultative physician including written report to requesting physician or other qualified health care professional, 5 minutes
99452	Interprofessional telephone/internet/electronic health record referral service(s) provided by a treating/requesting physician or other qualified health care professional, 30 minutes
Online/digital codes not included in analyses	
98969	Online evaluation and management service provided by a qualified non-physician health care professional to an established patient, guardian or health care provider not originating from a related assessment and management service provided within the previous 7 days, using the Internet or similar electronic communications network.
98970	Qualified nonphysician health care professional online digital evaluation and management service, for an established patient, for up to 7 days, cumulative time during the 7 days: 5–10 minutes
98971	11–20 minutes
98972	21–30 minutes
99444	Online evaluation and management service provided by a physician to an established patient, guardian or health care provider not originating from a related E&M service provided within the previous 7 days, using the Internet or similar electronic communications network.
99421	Online digital evaluation and management service, [physician or qualified health care professional] for an established patient, for up to 7 days cumulative time during the 7 days: 5–10 minutes
99422	11–20 minutes
99423	21–30 minutes
G2061	Qualified nonphysician healthcare professional online assessment and management service, for an established patient, for up to seven days, cumulative time during the 7 days; 5–10 minutes.
G2062	11–20 minutes
G2063	More than 20 minutes

NOTE: Table includes codes that are used for telehealth by a variety of providers, and some included in this list are not used in BH care. EEG = electroencephalogram.

Behavioral Health Utilization

This appendix presents data on monthly outpatient BH visits among service members with a diagnosis of PTSD, depression, or SUD in 2018–2020 (Figure B.1). Results are also shown by primary diagnosis (PTSD, depression, and SUD in Tables B.2–B.4). These results provide context for the analyses of the April–September 2019 and April–September 2020 periods.

FIGURE B.1

Number of Visits with Any BH Diagnosis Among Service Members with PTSD, Depression, or SUD, by Month, 2018–2020

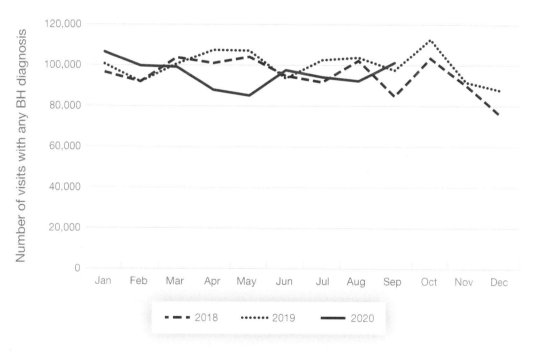

NOTE: Outpatient visits by month coded with a BH diagnosis in any position.

FIGURE B.2

Number of Visits with a PTSD Diagnosis Among Service Members with a Diagnosis of PTSD, Depression, or SUD, by Month, 2018–2020

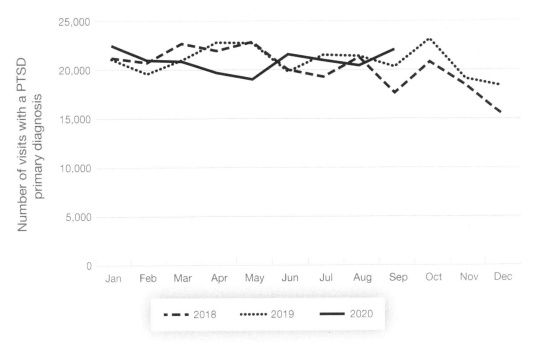

NOTE: Outpatient visits by month coded with PTSD in primary position.

FIGURE B.3

Number of Visits with a Depression Diagnosis Among Service Members with a Diagnosis of PTSD, Depression, or SUD, by Month, 2018–2020

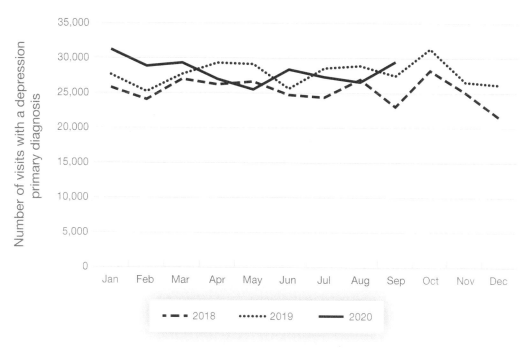

NOTE: Outpatient visits by month coded with depression in primary position.

Number of Visits with an SUD Diagnosis Among Service Members with a Diagnosis of PTSD, Depression, or SUD, by Month, 2018–2020

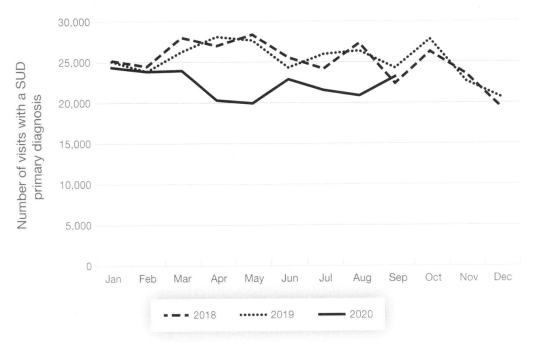

NOTE: Outpatient visits by month coded with SUD in primary position.

TABLE B.1

Number of BH Visits Within Three Months Among Service Members Initiating Care, by Diagnosis, 2019 and 2020

| | Number of BH Care Visits | | | | | | | |
| | April–September 2019 (%) | | | | April–September 2020 (%) | | | |
NTE Cohort	1	2–3	4–6	7+	1	2–3	4–6	7+
PTSD	(n = 1,807)				(n = 1,605)			
Any BH diagnosis, any position***	15.8	20.5	26.3	37.5	11.7	17.1	25.2	46.1
PTSD diagnosis, primary position***	27.1	24.0	24.5	24.4	22.8	20.8	23.9	32.5
Depression	(n = 4,525)				(n = 3,396)			
Any BH diagnosis, any position**	15.2	21.9	25.2	37.6	15.2	21.5	22.1	41.2
Depression diagnosis, primary position**	35.1	26.9	19.3	18.8	35.6	24.3	18.6	21.5
SUD	(n = 5,944)				(n = 4,672)			
Any BH diagnosis, any position***	19.9	14.6	13.9	49.5	17.5	14.7	15.1	49.6
SUD diagnosis, primary position***	16.7	11.5	10.9	33.7	15.5	12.4	13.3	31.0

NOTE: ** $p < 0.01$, *** $p < 0.001$.

TABLE B.2

Number of BH Visits Within Three Months Among Service Members Initiating Care and with One or More Visits, by Diagnosis and Visit Type, 2019 and 2020

| | Number of BH Care Visits | | | | | | | | | |
| | April–September 2019 (%) | | | | | April–September 2020 (%) | | | | |
NTE Cohort and Visit Type	*n*	1	2–3	4–6	7+	*n*	1	2–3	4–6	7+
PTSD										
Individual psychotherapy***	1,315	18.9	28.8	29.8	22.5	1,216	15.0	24.3	29.2	31.5
Group psychotherapy	87	32.2	31.0	17.2	19.5	33	45.5	18.2	18.2	18.2
E&M/medication management	834	54.7	32.9	9.4	3.1	670	47.8	38.8	10.2	3.3
Depression										
Individual psychotherapy***	2,665	25.9	32.7	24.4	16.9	1,985	24.6	26.2	25.3	23.9
Group psychotherapy	219	37.9	26.5	24.7	11.0	45	37.8	17.8	20.0	24.4
E&M/medication management	2,478	46.0	38.4	12.4	3.2	1,740	46.7	37.9	11.4	4.0
SUD										
Individual psychotherapy***	3,177	25.5	31.2	25.2	18.1	2,622	24.9	24.5	24.9	25.7
Group psychotherapy*	1,694	16.9	21.4	28.2	33.5	631	22.4	20.6	26.9	30.1
E&M/medication management	2,750	47.8	31.4	14.1	6.8	2,122	47.9	31.0	13.2	7.9

NOTE: * $p < 0.05$, *** $p < 0.001$.

Telehealth Utilization

When we examined how telehealth was coded (e.g., use of CPT-code modifiers and CPT codes that are specific to telephone telehealth) in April–September 2020, we saw apparent differences between direct and private-sector care in the coding used to document telehealth BH visits (Table C.1). Of the 291,439 telehealth visits in April–September 2020, 214,102 (73.5 percent) occurred in a direct care setting and 77,337 (26.5 percent) occurred in a private-sector care setting. Most telehealth visits during the six-month observation period in 2020 were audio-only and delivered by a direct care provider. In contrast, video telehealth accounted for the largest proportion of telehealth delivered by private-sector providers. Use of asynchronous telehealth was minimal in both direct and private-sector care (a total of 920 visits), which was not surprising, given our focus on BH care. Most audio-only visits in direct care settings were coded with CPT-code modifiers (e.g., T2025, G2012), in contrast to private-sector care, where those modifiers were not used.

TABLE C.1

Modalities of Coded BH Telehealth Visits Among Service Members with PTSD, Depression, or SUD, by Source of Care, April–September 2020

Modality	Total		Direct Care		Private-Sector Care	
	%	n	%	n	%	n
Video/synchronous (code with modifier)[a]	38.7	112,912	17.2	36,932	98.2	75,980
Asynchronous (code with modifier)[b]	0.3	920	0.2	452	0.6	468
Audio only/telephone (code with modifier)[c]	48.3	140,662	65.7	140,662	—	0
Audio only/telephone (CPT code)[d]	12.7	36,945	16.8	36,056	1.1	889
Total	100.0	291,439	100.0	214,102	100.0	77,337

[a] No telephone code AND modifier GT or 95 or MTF telehealth hub or place of service = 2.

[b] No telephone code AND modifier GQ or G2010.

[c] Modifier T2025 or G2012.

[d] 99441–99443, 98966–98968

We also examined the use of the six CPT codes documenting telephone E&M visits (99441–99443, 98966–98968) with a duration of 5–10 minutes, 11–20 minutes, or 21–30 minutes (Table C.2). In direct care, average monthly visits of this type most often involved a physician and were 5–10 minutes in duration, and monthly averages were similar in 2019 and 2020. There was some increase in average monthly visits for calls of longer duration. In contrast, these CPT-telephone E&M codes were not used at all in private-sector care in April–September 2019, and they were used minimally in the same months of 2020. These variations could reflect differences in the telehealth modalities used by direct and private-sector care providers or differences in the how the same telehealth modalities were coded.

TABLE C.2

Average Monthly Telephone E&M BH Visits for Service Members with PTSD, Depression, or SUD, by Source of Care, Provider Type, and Duration, 2019 and 2020

Source of Care	Duration of Telephone E&M BH Visits					
	Physician/Qualified Health Professional (mean number of visits)			Non-Physician (mean number of visits)		
	5–10 Minutes	11–20 Minutes	21–30 Minutes	5–10 Minutes	11–20 Minutes	21–30 Minutes
Direct care						
April–September 2019	5,860	159	72	232	40	17
April–September 2020	5,194	311	172	237	66	30
Private-sector care						
April–September 2019	0	0	0	0	0	0
April–September 2020	24	47	50	< 10	< 10	15

Quality Measure Scores and Telephone E&M Codes

For many quality measures used in this study, specifications for the numerator included specific CPT codes (e.g., psychotherapy, E&M for new or established patient). These codes stand alone, and we incorporated them into our measure scoring regardless of whether the care was delivered in person or via telehealth (i.e., with or without a telehealth modifier attached to the CPT code).

CPT codes for telephone E&M services of varying duration (5–30 minutes; CPT codes 99441–99443, 98966–98968) are a more recent addition to the list of telehealth visits that qualify as appropriate follow-up care as an acceptable alternative to in-person care (National Committee for Quality Assurance, undated). In applying the quality measures to both our 2019 and 2020 observations periods, we included these telephone E&M codes when the measure required a follow-up encounter and when the service was provided by an appropriate provider as dictated by the specific measure. We computed measure scores for both observation periods with and without this additional form of follow-up via telehealth (Table D.1).

When we did not include these codes in our analyses, applicable measure scores in April–September 2020 decreased by as much as 13 percent for follow-up after initiation of medication for AUD; by 4–7 percent for follow-up after new medication for PTSD, depression, or OUD; and by 1–2 percent for other measures, such as follow-up after an inpatient psychiatric hospitalization and MH- and AOD-related ED visits. When we similarly computed scores for the April–September 2019 observation period, we found that the same scores that did not include the telephone E&M CPT codes showed no change or a smaller decrease than those in 2020, reflecting, in part, the less frequent use of these codes in April–September 2019. The data presented here reflect the use of six E&M telephone codes and do not include details of telehealth coded by other means (e.g., CPT modifiers).

TABLE D.1
Selected Quality Measure Scores Computed with and Without Telephone E&M Codes, 2019 and 2020

Measure	April–September 2019			April–September 2020		
	Denominator	With Telephone E&M (%)	Without Telephone E&M (%)	Denominator	With Telephone E&M (%)	Without Telephone E&M (%)
Initial care						
PTSD: Receipt of care in first 8 weeks	2,464	28.5	27.4	2,261	35.8	34.1
DEP: Receipt of care in first 8 weeks	5,799	23.3	21.6	4,571	27.0	24.9
SUD: Engagement in treatment in 30 days	9,947	7.3	7.0	8,259	8.2	7.9
Medication management						
PTSD, new medication: E&M in 30 days	2,500	43.7	39.2	2,305	39.5	32.5
DEP, new medication: E&M in 30 days	7,024	42.0	38.2	6,315	39.5	34.2
AUD, new medication: E&M in 30 days	1,032	43.6	34.2	914	43.2	29.9
OUD, new medication: E&M in 30 days	211	14.2	11.4	129	11.6	7.8
Transitions of care						
Follow-up after MH hospitalization: 7 days	4,955	80.9	77.4	3,977	79.8	74.7
Follow-up after MH hospitalization: 30 days	4,955	91.9	90.9	3,977	90.0	88.3
Follow-up after ED for MH: 7 days	1,980	53.3	51.9	1,576	54.2	52.9
Follow-up after ED for MH: 30 days	1,980	68.8	67.7	1,576	69.2	68.1
Follow-up after ED for AOD: 7 days	884	16.9	16.1	622	23.3	22.0
Follow-up after ED for AOD: 30 days	884	25.6	24.3	622	35.0	33.6

NOTES: The columns labeled "With Telephone E&M" show measure scores computed with the option for telephone E&M lasting 5–30 minutes (CPT codes 99441–99443, 98966–98968) with an appropriate provider (as indicated by the quality measure). The "Without Telephone E&M" columns show measure scores computed without the option for telephone E&M lasting 5–30 minutes (CPT codes 99441–99443, 98966–98968) with an appropriate provider (as indicated by the quality measure).

Abbreviations

AOD	alcohol or other substance use disorder
AUD	alcohol use disorder
BH	behavioral health
BHDP	Behavioral Health Data Portal
COVID-19	coronavirus disease 2019
CPG	clinical practice guideline
CPT	Current Procedural Terminology
DHA	Defense Health Agency
DHHS	U.S. Department of Health and Human Services
DoD	U.S. Department of Defense
E&M	evaluation and management
ED	emergency department
FY	fiscal year
HCPCS	Healthcare Common Procedure Coding System
HIPAA	Health Insurance Portability and Accountability Act
ICD-10	International Classification of Diseases, 10th revision
MH	mental health
MHS	Military Health System
MTF	military treatment facility
NQF	National Quality Forum
NTE	new treatment episode
OUD	opioid use disorder
PTSD	posttraumatic stress disorder
SNRI	serotonin-norepinephrine update inhibitor
SSRI	selective serotonin reuptake inhibitor
SUD	substance use disorder
VA	U.S. Department of Veterans Affairs

References

Accountable Health Partners, "Excellus BlueCross BlueShield Code Guidance for Most Common Telehealth Services," April 28, 2020. As of January 13, 2022: https://ahpnetwork.com/wp-content/uploads/2020/04/EXC_TelehealthCOVID-19CodingGrid_revised4.28.2020.pdf

Aker, Janet A., "Military Health System Transformation Will Improve Care and Innovation," Military Health System, July 6, 2021. As of January 13, 2022: https://www.health.mil/News/Articles/2021/07/06/Military-Health-System-Transformation-Will-Improve-Care--Innovation

Alverson, Dale C., Karen Edison, Larry Flournoy, Brenda Korte, Charles Magruder, and Craig Miller, "Telehealth Tools for Public Health, Emergency, or Disaster Preparedness and Response: A Summary Report," *Telemedicine and E-Health*, Vol. 16, No. 1, January–February 2010, pp. 112–114.

American Telemedicine Association, *2017 GAPS Report: Coverage and Reimbursement*, Arlington, Va., October 2017.

Backhaus, Autumn, Zia Agha, Melissa L. Maglione, Andrea Repp, Bridgett Ross, Danielle Zuest, Natalie M. Rice-Thorp, James Lohr, and Steven R. Thorp, "Videoconferencing Psychotherapy: A Systematic Review," *Psychological Services*, Vol. 9, No. 2, May 2012, pp. 111–131.

Baer, Lee, D. Roderick Elford, and Peter Cukor, "Telepsychiatry at Forty: What Have We Learned?" *Harvard Review of Psychiatry*, Vol. 5, No. 1, May–June 1997, pp. 7–17.

Bashshur, Rashid L., Gary W. Shannon, Brian R. Smith, Dale C. Alverson, Nina Antoniotti, William G. Barsan, Noura Bashshur, Edward M. Brown, Molly J. Coye, Charles R. Doarn, et al., "The Empirical Foundations of Telemedicine Interventions for Chronic Disease Management," *Telemedicine and E-Health*, Vol. 20, No. 9, September 2014, pp. 769–800.

Breslau, Joshua, Melissa L. Finucane, Alicia R. Locker, Matthew D. Baird, Elizabeth A. Roth, and Rebecca L. Collins, "A Longitudinal Study of Psychological Distress in the United States Before and During the COVID-19 Pandemic," *Preventive Medicine*, Vol. 143, February 2021, article 106362.

Center for Connected Health Policy, "What Is Telehealth?" webpage, undated. As of January 13, 2022: https://www.cchpca.org/what-is-telehealth

Centers for Medicare and Medicaid Services, "President Trump Expands Telehealth Benefits for Medicare Beneficiaries During COVID-19 Outbreak," press release, March 17, 2020. As of January 13, 2022: https://www.cms.gov/newsroom/press-releases/president-trump-expands-telehealth-benefits-medicare-beneficiaries-during-covid-19-outbreak

Cohen, Gregory H., David S. Fink, Laura Sampson, and Sandro Galea, "Mental Health Among Reserve Component Military Service Members and Veterans," *Epidemiologic Reviews*, Vol. 37, No. 1, 2015, pp. 7–22.

Connolly, Samantha L., Leonie H. Stolzmann, Leonie Heyworth, Kendra R. Weaver, Mark S. Bauer, and Christopher J. Miller, "Rapid Increase in Telemental Health Within the Department of Veterans Affairs During the COVID-19 Pandemic," *Telemedicine and E-Health*, Vol. 27, No. 4, April 2021, pp. 454–458.

Cordts, Paul R., Defense Health Agency, "Interim Virtual Health (VH) Guidance During COVID-19 Pandemic Response," memorandum to market directors, Falls Church, Va., August 8, 2020.

Czeisler, Mark É., Rashon I. Lane, Joshua F. Wiley, Charles A. Czeisler, Mark E. Howard, and Shantha M. W. Rajaratnam, "Follow-Up Survey of US Adult Reports of Mental Health, Substance Use, and Suicidal Ideation During the COVID-19 Pandemic, September 2020," *JAMA Network Open*, Vol. 4, No. 2, February 1, 2021, article e2037665.

Defense Health Agency, "Interim Virtual Encounter Guidance During COVID-19 National Emergency," March 18, 2020.

Deshpande, Amol, Shariq Khoja, Julio Lorca, Ann McKibbon, Carlos Rizo, Donald Husereau, and Alejandro R. Jadad, "Asynchronous Telehealth: A Scoping Review of Analytic Studies," *Open Medicine*, Vol. 3, No. 2, June 2, 2009, pp. e69–e91.

DHA—*See* Defense Health Agency.

DHHS—*See* U.S. Department of Health and Human Services.

DoD—*See* U.S. Department of Defense.

Drug Enforcement Administration, "DEA Policy: Use of Telephone Evaluations to Initiate Buprenorphine Prescribing (Effective March 31, 2020)," memorandum, March 31, 2020. As of January 13, 2022:
https://www.deadiversion.usdoj.gov/coronavirus.html

Ettman, Catherine K., Salma M. Abdalla, Gregory H. Cohen, Laura Sampson, Patrick M. Vivier, and Sandro Galea, "Prevalence of Depression Symptoms in US Adults Before and During the COVID-19 Pandemic," *JAMA Network Open*, Vol. 3, No. 9, September 2, 2020, article e2019686.

Fortney, John C., Jeffrey M. Pyne, Timothy A. Kimbrell, Teresa J. Hudson, Dean E. Robinson, Ronald Schneider, William M. Moore, Paul J. Custer, Kathleen M. Grubbs, and Paula P. Schnurr, "Telemedicine-Based Collaborative Care for Posttraumatic Stress Disorder: A Randomized Clinical Trial," *JAMA Psychiatry*, Vol. 72, No. 1, January 2015, pp. 58–67.

Gentry, Melanie T., Maria I. Lapid, Matthew M. Clark, and Teresa A. Rummans, "Evidence for Telehealth Group-Based Treatment: A Systematic Review," *Journal of Telemedicine and Telecare*, Vol. 25, No. 6, July 2019, pp. 327–342.

Health Net Federal Services, "Telemedicine Billing Tips," webpage, undated. As of January 13, 2022:
https://www.tricare-west.com/content/hnfs/home/tw/prov/claims/billing_tips/telemedicine.html

Hepner, Kimberly A., Ryan Andrew Brown, Carol P. Roth, Teague Ruder, and Harold Alan Pincus, *Behavioral Health Care in the Military Health System: Access and Quality for Remote Service Members*, Santa Monica, Calif.: RAND Corporation, RR-2788-OSD, 2021. As of January 13, 2022:
https://www.rand.org/pubs/research_reports/RR2788.html

Hepner, Kimberly A., Carol P. Roth, Elizabeth M. Sloss, Susan M. Paddock, Praise O. Iyiewuare, Martha J. Timmer, and Harold Alan Pincus, *Quality of Care for PTSD and Depression in the Military Health System: Final Report*, Santa Monica, Calif.: RAND Corporation, RR-1542-OSD, 2017. As of January 13, 2022:
https://www.rand.org/pubs/research_reports/RR1542.html

Hepner, Kimberly A., Elizabeth M. Sloss, Carol P. Roth, Heather Krull, Susan M. Paddock, Shaela Moen, Martha J. Timmer, and Harold Alan Pincus, *Quality of Care for PTSD and Depression in the Military Health System: Phase I Report*, Santa Monica, Calif.: RAND Corporation, RR-978-OSD, 2016. As of January 13, 2022:
https://www.rand.org/pubs/research_reports/RR978.html

Hepner, Kimberly A., Jessica L. Sousa, Justin Hummer, Harold Alan Pincus, and Ryan Andrew Brown, *Military Behavioral Health Staff Perspectives on Telehealth Following the Onset of the COVID-19 Pandemic*, Santa Monica, Calif.: RAND Corporation, RR-A421-2, 2021. As of January 13, 2022:
https://www.rand.org/pubs/research_reports/RRA421-2.html

Hilty, Donald M., Daphne C. Ferrer, Michelle Burke Parish, Barb Johnston, Edward J. Callahan, and Peter M. Yellowlees, "The Effectiveness of Telemental Health: A 2013 Review," *Telemedicine and E-Health*, Vol. 19, No. 6, June 2013, pp. 444–454.

Holland, Kristin M., Christopher Jones, Alana M. Vivolo-Kantor, Nimi Idaikkadar, Marissa Zwald, Brooke Hoots, Ellen Yard, Ashley D'Inverno, Elizabeth Swedo, May S. Chen, et al., "Trends in US Emergency Department Visits for Mental Health, Overdose, and Violence Outcomes Before and During the COVID-19 Pandemic," *JAMA Psychiatry*, Vol. 78, No. 4, April 1, 2021, pp. 372–379.

Humana Military, "Coronavirus Disease (COVID-19) and TRICARE's Telemedicine Benefit," April 29, 2020. As of January 13, 2022:
https://www.humanamilitary.com/provider/education-and-resources/quick-access/policy-updates-and-alerts/COVID-19-telemedicine-031320

Hummer, Justin, Kimberly A. Hepner, Carol P. Roth, Ryan Andrew Brown, Jessica L. Sousa, Teague Ruder, and Harold Alan Pincus, *Behavioral Health Care for National Guard and Reserve Service Members from the Military Health System*, Santa Monica, Calif.: RAND Corporation, RR-A421-1, 2021. As of January 13, 2022:
https://www.rand.org/pubs/research_reports/RRA421-1.html

Jowers, Karen, "Are Military Patients Delaying the Health Care They Need?" *Military Times*, May 13, 2020. As of January 13, 2022:
https://www.militarytimes.com/pay-benefits/2020/05/13/are-military-patients-delaying-the-health-care-they-need

Kime, Patricia, "MOAA's 2020–21 TRICARE Guide: Is Telehealth Here to Stay?" Military Officers Association of America, December 4, 2020. As of January 13, 2022:
https://www.moaa.org/content/publications-and-media/news-articles/2020-news-articles/moaas-2020-21-tricare-guide-is-telehealth-here-to-stay

Lin, Lewei Allison, Anne C. Fernandez, and Erin E. Bonar, "Telehealth for Substance-Using Populations in the Age of Coronavirus Disease 2019: Recommendations to Enhance Adoption," *JAMA Psychiatry*, Vol. 77, No. 12, December 1, 2020, pp. 1209–1210.

Lurie, Nicole, and Brendan G. Carr, "The Role of Telehealth in the Medical Response to Disasters," *JAMA Internal Medicine*, Vol. 178, No. 6, June 2018, pp. 745–746.

Luxton, David D., Larry D. Pruitt, Karen O'Brien, and Gregory Kramer, "An Evaluation of the Feasibility and Safety of a Home-Based Telemental Health Treatment for Posttraumatic Stress in the U.S. Military," *Telemedicine and E-Health*, Vol. 21, No. 11, November 2015, pp. 880–886.

Luxton, David D., Larry D. Pruitt, Amy Wagner, Derek J. Smolenski, Michael A. Jenkins-Guarnieri, and Gregory Gahm, "Home-Based Telebehavioral Health for U.S. Military Personnel and Veterans with Depression: A Randomized Controlled Trial," *Journal of Consulting and Clinical Psychology*, Vol. 84, No. 11, November 2016, pp. 923–934.

Madsen, Cathaleen, Amanda Banaag, and Tracey Pérez Koehlmoos, "Analysis of Telehealth Usage and Trends in the Military Health System, 2006–2018," *Telemedicine and E-Health*, Vol. 27, No. 12, December 2021.

Mann, Devin M., Ji Chen, Rumi Chunara, Paul A. Testa, and Oded Nov, "COVID-19 Transforms Health Care Through Telemedicine: Evidence from the Field," *Journal of the American Medical Informatics Association*, Vol. 27, No. 7, July 1, 2020, pp. 1132–1135.

McGinty, Emma E., Rachel Presskreischer, Hahrie Han, and Colleen L. Barry, "Psychological Distress and Loneliness Reported by US Adults in 2018 and April 2020," *JAMA*, Vol. 324, No. 1, June 3, 2020, pp. 93–94.

Mehrotra, Ateev, Michael Chernew, David Linetsky, Hilary Hatch, and David A. Cutler, "The Impact of the COVID-19 Pandemic on Outpatient Visits: A Rebound Emerges," blog post, Commonwealth Fund, May 19, 2020. As of January 26, 2021: https://www.commonwealthfund.org/publications/2020/apr/impact-covid-19-outpatient-visits

Mehrotra, Ateev, Michael E. Chernew, David Linetsky, Hilary Hatch, David A. Cutler, and Eric C. Schneider, *The Impact of COVID-19 on Outpatient Visits in 2020: Visits Remained Stable, Despite a Late Surge in Cases*, New York: Commonwealth Fund, February 22, 2021. As of January 13, 2022: https://www.commonwealthfund.org/publications/2021/feb/ impact-covid-19-outpatient-visits-2020-visits-stable-despite-late-surge

MHS—*See* Military Health System.

Military Health System, "Frequently Asked Questions: Telehealth," webpage, undated. As of May 11, 2022: https://www.health.mil/Reference-Center/Frequently-Asked-Questions/Telehealth

———, "Frequently Asked Questions: COVID-19 and Virtual Health for Providers," fact sheet, June 1, 2020.

Military Health System Communications Office, "MTFs Respond to COVID-19 with Increased Telehealth, Drive-Thrus," December 29, 2020. As of January 13, 2022: https://www.health.mil/News/Articles/2020/12/29/MTFs-respond-to-COVID-19-with-increased-telehealth-drive-thrus

National Capital Consortium Pediatrics, "Telemedicine Cheat Sheet," April 22, 2020.

National Center for Health Statistics, "Early Release of Selected Mental Health Estimates Based on Data from the January–June 2019 National Health Interview Survey," May 2020. As of January 13, 2022: https://www.cdc.gov/nchs/data/nhis/earlyrelease/ERmentalhealth-508.pdf

National Committee for Quality Assurance, "Follow-Up After Hospitalization for Mental Illness (FUH)," webpage, undated. As of January 13, 2022: https://www.ncqa.org/hedis/measures/follow-up-after-hospitalization-for-mental-illness

National Quality Forum, homepage, undated. As of January 13, 2022: https://www.qualityforum.org/Home.aspx

Olthuis, Janine V., Lori Wozney, Gordon J. G. Asmundson, Heidi Cramm, Patricia Lingley-Pottie, and Patrick J. McGrath, "Distance-Delivered Interventions for PTSD: A Systematic Review and Meta-Analysis," *Journal of Anxiety Disorders*, Vol. 44, December 2016, pp. 9–26.

Pamplin, Jeremy C., Konrad L. Davis, Jennifer Mbuthia, Steven Cain, Sean J. Hipp, Daniel J. Yourk, Christopher J. Colombo, and Ron Poropatich, "Military Telehealth: A Model for Delivering Expertise to the Point of Need in Austere and Operational Environments," *Health Affairs (Millwood)*, Vol. 38, No. 8, August 2019, pp. 1386–1392.

Patel, Sadiq Y., Ateev Mehrotra, Haiden A. Huskamp, Lori Uscher-Pines, Ishani Ganguli, and Michael L. Barnett, "Trends in Outpatient Care Delivery and Telemedicine During the COVID-19 Pandemic in the US," *JAMA Internal Medicine*, Vol. 181, No. 3, November 16, 2020, pp. 388–391.

Place, Ronald J., Defense Health Agency, "Tiered Telehealth Health Care Support for COVID-19," memorandum to market directors, Falls Church, Va., March 27, 2020.

Public Law 114-328, National Defense Authorization Act for Fiscal Year 2017, December 23, 2016.

Rosen, Craig S., Leslie A. Morland, Lisa H. Glassman, Brian P. Marx, Kendra Weaver, Clifford A. Smith, Stacey Pollack, and Paula P. Schnurr, "Virtual Mental Health Care in the Veterans Health Administration's Immediate Response to Coronavirus Disease–19," *American Psychologist*, Vol. 76, No. 1, January 2021, pp. 26–38.

Shigekawa, Erin, Margaret Fix, Garen Corbett, Dylan H. Roby, and Janet Coffman, "The Current State of Telehealth Evidence: A Rapid Review," *Health Affairs (Millwood)*, Vol. 37, No. 12, December 2018, pp. 1975–1982.

Smith, Anthony C., Emma Thomas, Centaine L. Snoswell, Helen Haydon, Ateev Mehrotra, Jane Clemensen, and Liam J. Caffery, "Telehealth for Global Emergencies: Implications for Coronavirus Disease 2019 (COVID-19)," *Journal of Telemedicine and Telecare*, Vol. 26, No. 5, June 2020, pp. 309–313.

Strong, Jessica, Jennifer Akin, and Drew Brazer, *Pain Points Poll Deep Dive: Understanding the Impact of COVID-19 on Mental Health*, Encinitas, Calif.: Blue Star Families, 2020. As of January 13, 2022:
https://bluestarfam.org/wp-content/uploads/2020/08/BSF-COVID-PPP-DeepDive-MentalHealth_ver2.pdf

Torous, John, and Til Wykes, "Opportunities from the Coronavirus Disease 2019 Pandemic for Transforming Psychiatric Care with Telehealth," *JAMA Psychiatry*, Vol. 77, No. 12, December 1, 2020, pp. 1205–1206.

Uscher-Pines, Lori, Jessica L. Sousa, Pushpa Raja, Ateev Mehrotra, Michael L. Barnett, and Haiden A. Huskamp, "Suddenly Becoming a 'Virtual Doctor': Experiences of Psychiatrists Transitioning to Telemedicine During the COVID-19 Pandemic," *Psychiatric Services*, Vol. 71, No. 11, November 1, 2020, pp. 1143–1150.

U.S. Department of Defense, "TRICARE Coverage and Payment for Certain Services in Response to the COVID-19 Pandemic," May 12, 2020. As of January 13, 2022:
https://www.federalregister.gov/documents/2020/05/12/2020-10042/tricare-coverage-and-payment-for-certain-services-in-response-to-the-covid-19-pandemic

———, "Coronavirus: Timeline," webpage, last updated January 12, 2022. As of January 13, 2022:
https://www.defense.gov/Spotlights/Coronavirus-DOD-Response/Timeline

U.S. Department of Health and Human Services, "Notification of Enforcement Discretion for Telehealth Remote Communications During the COVID-19 Nationwide Public Health Emergency," April 21, 2020. As of January 13, 2022:
https://www.federalregister.gov/documents/2020/04/21/2020-08416/notification-of-enforcement-discretion-for-telehealth-remote-communications-during-the-covid-19

————, "Public Health Emergency Declarations," webpage, last updated January 7, 2022. As of January 13, 2022:
https://www.phe.gov/emergency/news/healthactions/phe/Pages/default.aspx

U.S. Department of Veterans Affairs and U.S. Department of Defense, *VA/DoD Clinical Practice Guideline for the Management of Substance Use Disorder*, version 3.0, December 2015. As of January 13, 2022:
https://www.healthquality.va.gov/guidelines/MH/sud/VADoDSUDCPGRevised22216.pdf

————, *VA/DoD Clinical Practice Guideline for the Management of Major Depressive Disorder*, version 3.0, Washington, D.C., April 2016.

————, *VA/DoD Clinical Practice Guideline for the Management of Posttraumatic Stress Disorder*, version 3.0, Washington, D.C., June 2017.

U.S. Government Accountability Office, *Department of Defense: Telehealth Use in Fiscal Year 2016*, Washington D.C., GAO-18-108R, November 14, 2017.

U.S. House of Representatives, *National Defense Authorization Act for Fiscal Year 2017 Conference Report to Accompany S. 2943*, 114th Congress, 2nd Session, Washington, D.C.: U.S. Government Publishing Office, Report 114-840, November 30, 2016.

VA—*See* U.S. Department of Veterans Affairs.

Vahratian, Anjel, Stephen J. Blumberg, Emily P. Terlizzi, and Jeannine S. Schiller, "Symptoms of Anxiety or Depressive Disorder and Use of Mental Health Care Among Adults During the COVID-19 Pandemic—United States, August 2020–February 2021," *Morbidity Mortality Weekly Report*, Vol. 70, No. 13, April 2, 2021, pp. 490–494.

Verma, Seema, "Early Impact of CMS Expansion of Medicare Telehealth During COVID-19," *Health Affairs Forefront*, July 15, 2020. As of January 13, 2022:
https://www.healthaffairs.org/do/10.1377/hblog20200715.454789/full

Volk, JoAnn, Dania Palanker, Madeline O'Brien, and Christina L. Goe, *States' Actions to Expand Telemedicine Access During COVID-19 and Future Policy Considerations*, New York: Commonwealth Fund, June 23, 2021. As of January 13, 2022:
https://www.commonwealthfund.org/publications/issue-briefs/2021/jun/states-actions-expand-telemedicine-access-covid-19

Wheeler, William, "Partnerships, COVID-19 Are Catalysts for Enterprise Virtual Health," U.S. Department of Defense, January 20, 2021. As of January 13, 2022:
https://www.defense.gov/News/Feature-Stories/Story/Article/2470534/partnerships-covid-19-are-catalysts-for-enterprise-virtual-health